FIT IN NO TIME

AXEL DELKER & LAURA SCHÖFFEL

FIT IN NO TIME

A STRONGER BACK IN ONE MINUTE A DAY

IMPRINT

1st edition 2020
© Axel Delker & Laura Schöffel
Am Gielbrunnen 3, 67304 Eisenberg,

Germany

Photographs
Lisa Beller with Lasse Schneider

Layout, typesetting and cover
schönski GmbH

Editing
Michelle Sattinger & Konstantin Hauck

Text
Laura Schöffel & Axel Delker

Concept
Axel Delker

Translation
Thomas D. Green

"We could have started a conspiracy against time."

CLAUDE LÉVI-STRAUSS

CONTENT

THE KEY

FIT IN NO TIME puts the key to a fitter life in your hands. This isn't just any key—it's a master key, the universal lock-pick of exercise programs. It fits for anyone and everyone. It opens the door to a healthier life for those who don't exercise. And for those who do, it improves the physical foundation for performance for everyone, whether amateur athlete or multiple Wimbledon champion.

Many of the pages that follow focus on getting started with exercise and building the fundamentals of fitness. This is what this workout is all about: it invites you to set out on your journey to a body that feels a whole lot better. And that's what this book is about: it's an invitation to make your life healthier without having to change it. FIT IN NO TIME is the result of my search for a workout that would fit into my daily schedule without requiring compromises, sacrifices or some other workaround to get it done.

Plagued by back problems at an early age, I found that conventional remedies such as physiotherapy and exercising in a gym did not offer me the relief I sought. Besides, all this just took up too much of my time.

So I set out on my own, searching from my perspective as an economist and impassioned pragmatist.

IT'S A MASTER KEY

I wanted the best results possible with limited resources. Time is the scarcest resource in my life, so I starting looking for answers with minutes in mind. This combination of making the most of the minutes I have to spare and drawing on the latest insights in sports science has proven its merits for many years. It makes my life healthier without leaving me even more pressed for time.

Sometimes big problems can be solved with simple means: One minute of training a day is enough for FIT IN NO TIME. And the 15 minutes you spend reading this book could pay dividends for many tomorrows to come.

In many countries, such as the US, Canada, Finland and Germany, back pain is the leading cause of mobility impairment and work disability.[1,2] This book aims to fix that issue and help a fitter you enjoy your days free of that pain.

So, where do we start? We have to pull this problem up by the roots, and those are in our minds and in our habits. We are all aware of the benefits of being active, but close to one in two adults in my country, Germany, hardly ever exercises.[3] The number in your country is probably similar.

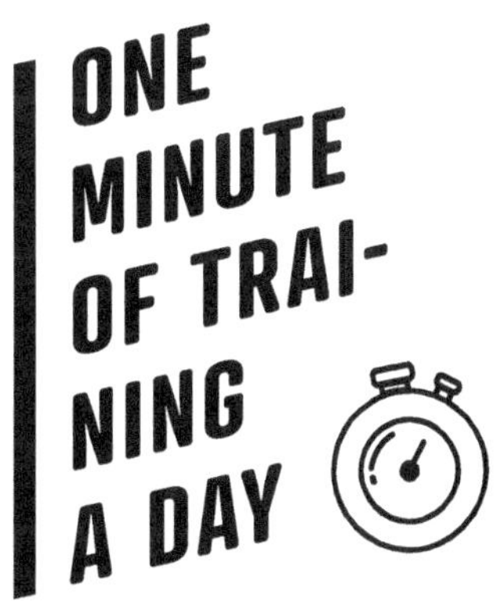

FIT IN NO TIME

takes this paradox and
runs with it:

CHAPTER 1 turns conventional fitness wisdom on its head and shows you why so many good intentions go awry and often end up taking us on a guilt trip.

I.

CHAPTER 2 shows that a daily one-minute workout really is enough for our purpose—if we do the right exercises!

II.

III.

CHAPTER 3 is all about getting you off to a good start. Read it and you will understand why the solution has always been as close at hand as your tooth-brush.

IV.

CHAPTER 4 wraps things up with a closer look at the workout and how to perform the exercises.

LET'S GET RIGHT TO IT.

Only 72 PAGES separate you from the beginnings of a fitter life and stronger back.

THE PROBLEM

FIT IN NO TIME was born of an encounter I had one evening after a long day at the office. That night, I headed to the gym more out of a sense of duty than any genuine desire, showing up at 10:59 p.m., a minute before the gym was to close. My trainer, busy packing his things and clearly annoyed, asked me, "What do you want? You can't get a workout in a minute." **That was a very good question, but how much truth was there to his follow-up statement?**

WHAT DO I WANT?

Finding out what we want isn't always easy. Thousands of books offer advice on decisions about this or that, some of which contradict each other. Getting our bearings is hard in a society that can't even agree on the compass points.[4,5] Setting and sticking to goals of your own in a world with so many conflicting influences takes some doing.

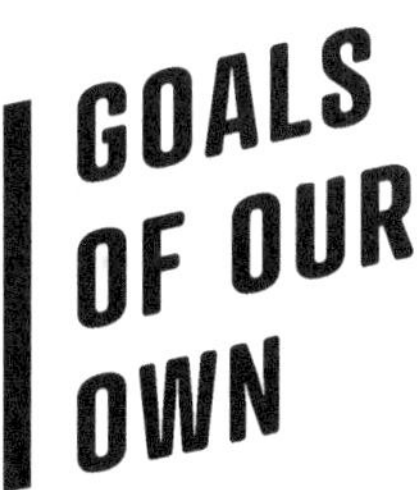

Your exercise goals are all your own. Where you want to go and how you aim to get there is for no one else to decide. The FIT IN NO TIME fitness pyramid provides orientation so you really can do it your way. It doesn't dictate goals, but it should help you stake out priorities and perhaps reconsider the order of your goals.

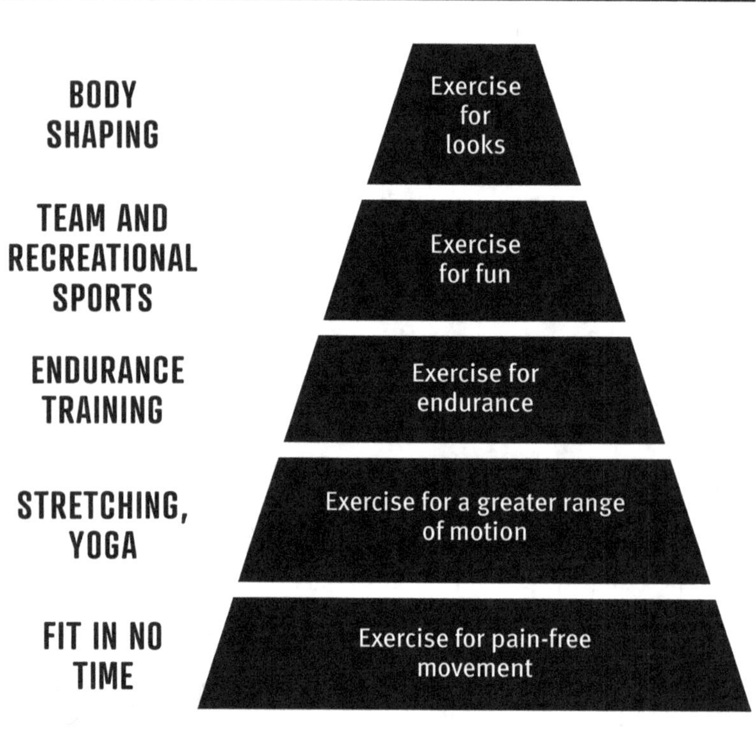

Again, back pain is the biggest inhibitor preventing people from enjoying everyday activities. This is where FIT IN NO TIME comes in. It puts within reach everything you need to make your day-to-day activity a pain-free experience. Any goal beyond that—a greater range of motion, more endurance or a body that looks a certain way—hinges on a healthy and strong back. If it hurts to move, we're not going to do it a lot or for long. This is why we start at the bottom of the pyramid to build resilient postural muscles in the back. Once that musculature is strong, you can move up the pyramid to pursue higher goals in a sustainable, healthy way.

If you don't exercise at all, FIT IN NO TIME gets you off to a healthy and fast start, building a foundation that will serve you well later. If you have already set higher goals for yourself, this workout will help you achieve them and maintain your gains over the long term.

A HEALTHY AND FAST START

The idea of progressive training sounds logical enough, but the reality of human nature defies that logic. How often have you seen people start training with very ambitious goals in mind? And how long are they able to hold themselves to those high expectations? Not long at all, sometimes. **And no matter how high you aim or how far you want to go, there is just no getting around a healthy foundation.**

HOW FAR WILL I GO?

"You can't get a workout in a minute." Is that true? Throughout our lives, we try to make the most of the resources we have at our disposal.[6] When we go to buy a car, take that annual vacation or shop for a new cell phone deal, we always look for the best option available on our budgets. In both our professional and personal lives, we measure our goals against the means at our disposal. But somehow these cost/benefit considerations just don't seem to figure into our fitness goals.

That certainly applies to me. I tried to achieve goals for which I simply did not have enough resources. In sports and fitness, the most valuable and decisive resource is time. Twice a week for one hour plus the trip to the gym—squeezing those demands into my weekly schedule didn't work for long.

Rather than accepting this reality, taking a step down the pyramid and aiming for more reasonable goals, I did something entirely unreasonable—I stopped working out altogether. For someone looking to buy a car, that's akin to saying *my budget won't stretch to a Mercedes, so I'll just walk.* Why not simply buy a Fiat instead?

If reports about the increasingly sedentary lifestyles in developed countries are true, then the old me wasn't the only couch potato thinking along these lines. Concerns about health and well-being are surely a factor in our growing awareness of the need for a more sustainable way of life and means of production, yet those same concerns haven't opened our minds to the idea of considering a resource-sparing exercise program. It hasn't occurred to us to question the notion that nothing less than an hour of training is going to work. This fallacy deserves some of the blame when we give up on our good intentions.

When we abandon our plans, we fail to realize that we can achieve a lot with just a little time and effort. What else would explain why nearly half my fellow Germans don't exercise at all? Surely everyone has a few minutes to spare.

I suggest that we look at exercise like any other of life's many transactions. Let's first take stock of our resources and then make the most of what we have. The question then is not *can I get a workout in a minute,* but rather *er how much of a workout can I get in a minute.*

THE MOVER MATRIX

Now let's plug the two big questions discussed earlier—*What do I want?* and *How far will I go?* into what I call the *mover matrix,* because it's all about what moves you to get moving.

This matrix illustrates the relationship between the time invested and the benefit obtained. It dispels any foggy notions we may have about time and effort.

Clearly, we have to invest more time for higher goals than for lower ones. There is just no way around that. It's so obvious, yet so many people do what I did for so long—they ignore that fitness fundamental. We reach for goals that demand hours of effort in the hope that a few minutes will do the trick.

I think we can all agree that 60 seconds of training a day is not going to put us on the cover of a fitness magazine or condition us to be elite tennis players. It takes a lot of practice to excel at a sport or instrument. The science would suggest that it takes around 10,000 hours on average to attain mastery.[7] Whatever the number may be for buff fitness models, it's not going to be measured in minutes.

In the *mover matrix*, I call this disconnect the *guilt triangle*. If we keep setting goals beyond our reach, we're setting ourselves up for constant failure. You may know that sinking feeling—it's all too familiar to me—and it usually hits hardest when we realize we're another monthly fee poorer for not having set foot in the gym.

But there's a way out of that guilt triangle: stick with the time that you can afford to put in, but step down your goal. You'll find yourself in a happier place, the feel-good triangle. It's a lot more gratifying when you know your effort will be sufficient for what you hope to achieve. Instead of aiming high for an hour's workout and feeling guilty about falling short, aim lower so just one minute of your time each day will let you achieve what you set out to do.

The message behind this matrix is that remarkable progress is indeed obtainable in a very short time if you pursue the right goals. Of course, there's a trick to achieving a lot with a little—it's called efficiency.

As fresh as this insight may be in the fitness world, it's not new to the real world. Back in the 19th century, the Italian economist Vilfredo Pareto came up with the 80/20 rule, which much of the world today knows as the Pareto principle. It states that 80 percent of a goal can be achieved with 20 percent resource input.[8] We can apply this rule to the *mover matrix* and the question of how to make the most of our resources to find out what constitutes t*he most efficient 20 percent input.*

In other words, we have to find the most efficient exercises—some form of workout that gets us fit for everyday activities with just 60 seconds of training a day.

FIND THE MOST EFFICIENT 20 %?

THE SOLUTION

THE MAGIC MINUTE

A minute can feel like a long time. Manchester United famously turned the tables on Bayern München in the 1999 Champions League final, snatching victory from the jaws of defeat in just one minute. The hundred-meter women and men's sprints are the banner events of every Summer Olympics. Those memorable ten seconds, give or take, leave an indelible impression on spectators. One of the most riveting events in modern German history took just two seconds: John F. Kennedy touched the hearts of millions with his celebrated "Ich bin ein Berliner." In truth, though, a minute is neither short nor long. Time is indeed relative[9] or, as Martin Luther King put it, "Time itself is neutral."[10] It is up to us to put time to good use, to do something meaningful with it that suits our purposes. It rolls on whether we take action or not; the minutes and years pass with nothing happening in and of time itself. Time doesn't care when you take a random minute of your morning and turn it into your magic minute—that decision is entirely up to you.

The science would seem to corroborate the premise that underpins the *mover matrix*. A 2014 study conducted by McMaster University in Canada found that a one-minute training session can achieve much the same effect as a thirty-minute workout.[11] There is a caveat, though: Athletes have to push themselves to their limit throughout its brief span for this training to work. Then it is extremely effective. Our muscles need this intense stimulus, the stress that comes with being put under a load, to grow regardless of the duration of the training.[12] To put it simply, the only way to grow stronger is to overload our muscles. This is the idea behind high-intensity training. And more and more scientific studies on the effects of exercise even suggest that people can improve their endurance with a one-minute program. This defies the conventional wisdom that endurance training has to be a long slog.[13] Compared to these more radical regimens, FIT IN NO TIME looks almost conservative. A one-minute workout of maximum intensity training achieves the desired aim, and FIT IN NO TIME takes advantage of that effect. **Simply jogging around the block for a minute or smacking a few golf balls is not going to do the trick.**

MAXIMUM INTENSITY

THE YIN & YANG OF A STRONG BACK

Our goal is to get in shape for everyday activities. For that, we need a strong back and an exercise regimen that puts all the postural muscle groups under a load and pushes them to the limit within 60 seconds.

This is all about fundamental fitness, so the regimen has to:

- be easy to learn
- require little in the way of equipment
- avoid muscle imbalances that cause or aggravate postural issues

That last point merits special attention. When we engage in strength training, we sometimes favor some exercises over others. Too much pushing and not enough pulling, or vice versa, can lead to muscle imbalances that throw our posture out of whack. This is why you have to challenge muscles in both directions of movement, exercising flexor and extensor muscle groups in equal measure.[12] Another important point to consider is rest. The muscle groups trained in one session deserve at least 24 hours rest, or better still, 48 hours. This gives the body time to react to the load placed on its muscles by stimulating growth.[12] If we fail to give muscles time to grow, training can have the opposite effect. Overloading muscles without proper rest tears them down instead of building them up.

How do you like the sound of that? Even if you train for just a minute a day, you still have to be careful not to overdo it.

FIT IN NO TIME factors rest into the exercise equation. Its effective, healthy training regimen consists of two classic and complementary exercises—chin-ups and push-ups performed on alternate days. Like the opposing forces of yin and yang, they interact to build a well-balanced foundation

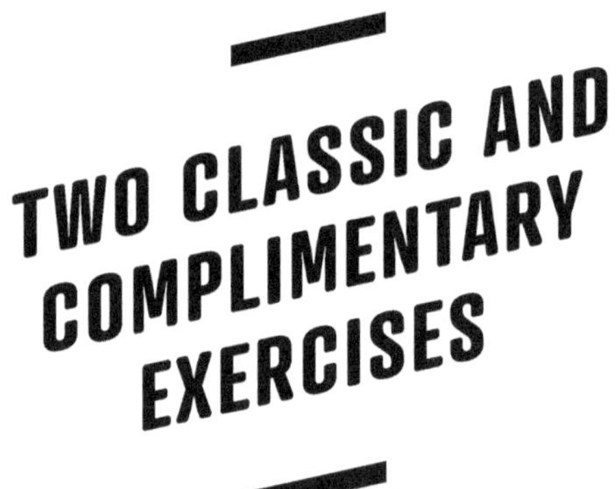

for your fitness.

You may be thinking, "Oh no, I can't do chin-ups." Let me put your concerns to rest: the tips and tricks found in CHAPTER 4 will have you well on your way to your first successful chin-up.

The chin-up is the silver bullet in the arsenal of resistance exercises. It trains the *latissimus dorsi*, one of the largest muscles in the body. Commonly called lats in the plural, this muscle stabilizes the lumbar spine and, by extension, the entire back. Attached to the humerus, it draws the upper arm downward toward the trunk. Lats also perform very important functions for the back. In combination with the deep lateral abdominal muscles, the back extensors and the superficial large gluteal muscle, they provide the muscular tension for the thoracolumbar fascia, or firm sheets of connective tissue seated deep in the lower back. This is the spinal column's main stabilizing system. It connects to all 24 movable vertebrae and the pelvis via several compartments. The chin-up also works many other muscles, including scapular (shoulder blade) retractors and depressors, muscles of the hand and forearm, back extensors, abdominal muscles and all arm flexors.[14,15] Hardly any other exercise builds muscles in the upper body as rapidly as the chin-up or addresses as many muscles at the same time. This is a huge advantage—the more muscle mass you activate, the more muscle-building hormones your body secretes.

The push-up is the perfect complement to the chin-up. Each exercise packs a punch, but the interaction between the two is a powerful one-two combination that can't be beat. The push-up's pressing action trains antagonist muscle groups— that is, the counterparts of the muscles worked by the chin-up's pulling action. Like the chin-up, it also trains many muscle groups in your chest, back, arms and torso. Unlike the chin-up, it also works your buttocks, called glutes in training vernacular.[16]

Performing just one exercise is a recipe for muscular imbalance. We have to alternate between the two to build a stable foundation for fitness. Another reason why these particular exercises lend themselves to FIT IN NO TIME is that each lets you train hard enough to exert yourself within a minute. As we learned earlier, that is the intensity science demands of us for an effective workout.

By combining the two exercises, we also meet the demands of that last point addressed above— rest. Alternating the two exercises, performing one today and the other tomorrow, automatically gives the muscle groups a long enough break for them to rest and recuperate. If you do chin-ups on Mondays and push-ups on Tuesdays, the muscle groups of the chin-up training can recover for 48 hours and are rested and ready for the next session on Wednesdays. The FIT IN NO TIME training journal on PAGE 68 will help you to maintain this rhythm. It also points you to new training stimuli when the introductory exercises in CHAPTER 4 no longer push you to your limit within a minute.

Now that you know what the exercises are and what the science says we need to do, let's focus on the most important thing—your mind.

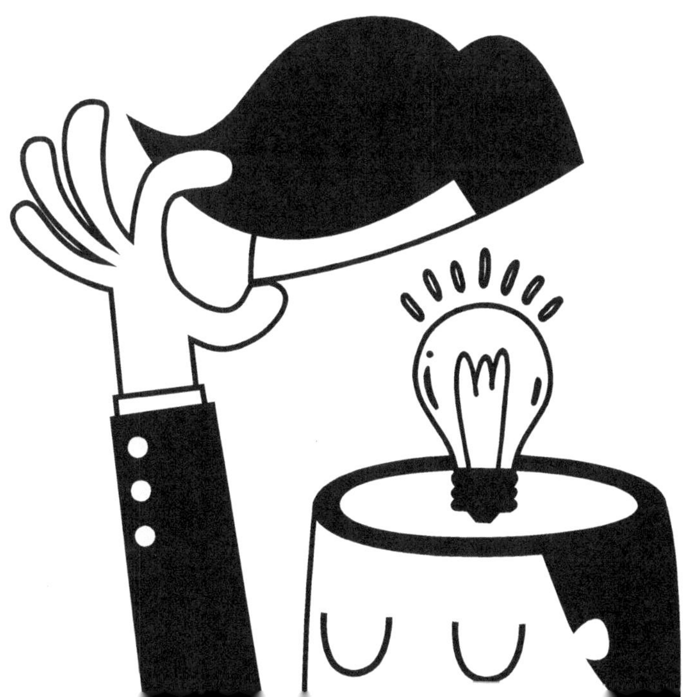

PRACTICAL APPLICATION

GETTING STARTED

I find that two things grease the gears when I start something new:

For one, you have to actually see and feel the need for change to create a sense of urgency. That idea stems from Professor John Kotter, an acknowledged change management expert.[17]

For the other, getting started has to be easy. The door needs to be open and the path to it free of obstacles. This is what economists mean by low entry barriers.[18]

As to how the first relates to my fitness journey, I saw the need for change and certainly felt the urgency of it. My wake-up call came soon after I graduated from university and started working. In my first year on the job, I suffered acute lumbago twice. An underdeveloped musculature and long periods of sitting are known to favor this sudden onset of sharp pain in the lumbar region. Just 25 years old, I had heard of this condition, but even my grandparents had never had anything like that. I was shocked that back problems had hit me so early and suddenly. One thought triggered an impending sense of urgency in me: *If it's as bad as this now, what am I going*

feel like when I'm 40 or 50, let alone 70 or 80?
Only you can know what sense of urgency motivates you. It may be as simple as the desire to get up and get moving. Perhaps you're keen to prevent back problems. Or maybe it's something completely different, but whatever it is, that motivation definitely has to come from within you.

YOUR SENSE OF URGENCY

I had seen and felt the need for change, but what I lacked was low entry barriers to training that would strengthen my back. Instead, it was my desire to relieve that pain that drove me to join a local gym, and to my trainer's now familiar utterance, "You can't get a workout in a minute."

FIT IN NO TIME was born of this situation. It puts the solution to the problem of low entry barriers at your fingertips.

The low entry barriers to the FIT IN NO TIME regimen owe a great deal to a survey[3] of couch potatoes and their most frequently stated reasons for eschewing physical activity. It's not that they don't feel the need to exercise—on the contrary, the lack of it is a heavy emotional burden for most people who make no effort to do their bodies a good turn. Asked why they choose not to engage in any physical activity, the majority of non-exercisers cited two mundane reasons for their involuntary abstinence: the lack of time and the prohibitively long trip to the venue.

Our one minute takes care of those reservations

about time, but we still don't have the right place for the workout.

My chin-up bar went up over the door to my shower. I step into it every day anyway, so I don't have to take any detours to get to the place I train. If there's any truth to that survey of non-exercisers, details like this can make all the difference.

My experience bears that out. Even small departures from the routine can sabotage your chin-up and push-up regimen. After moving house, I put the chin-up bar in my basement office. It was just a few steps down the stairs, but that detour was enough to

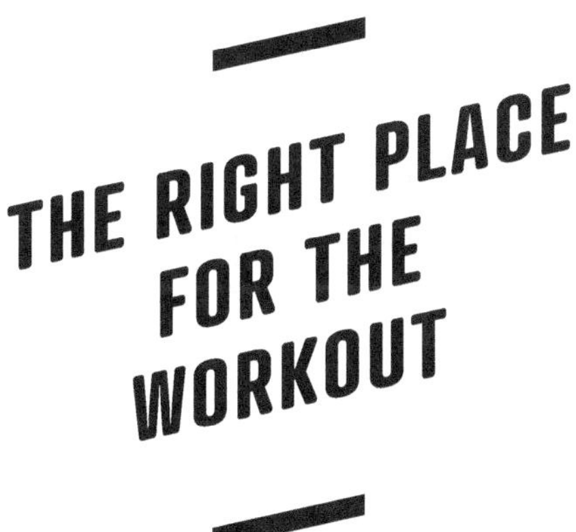

inspire me to come up with this or that excuse to say "not today."

This taught me an important lesson: Every extra meter and increment of time can put distance between you and your training and make it so much easier to say "not today"—especially in the morning. **Don't underestimate that when choosing the right place to put your chin-up bar.**

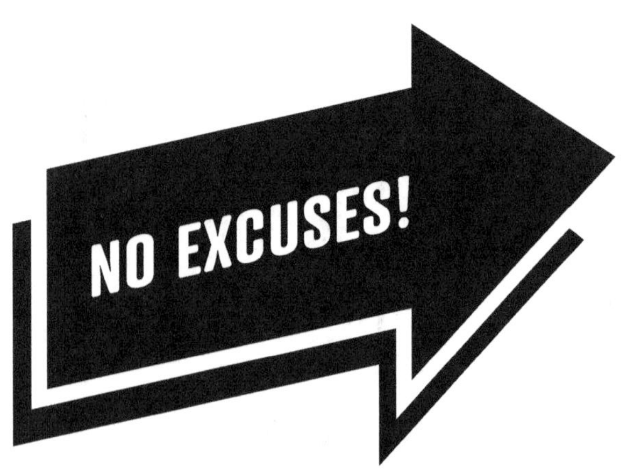

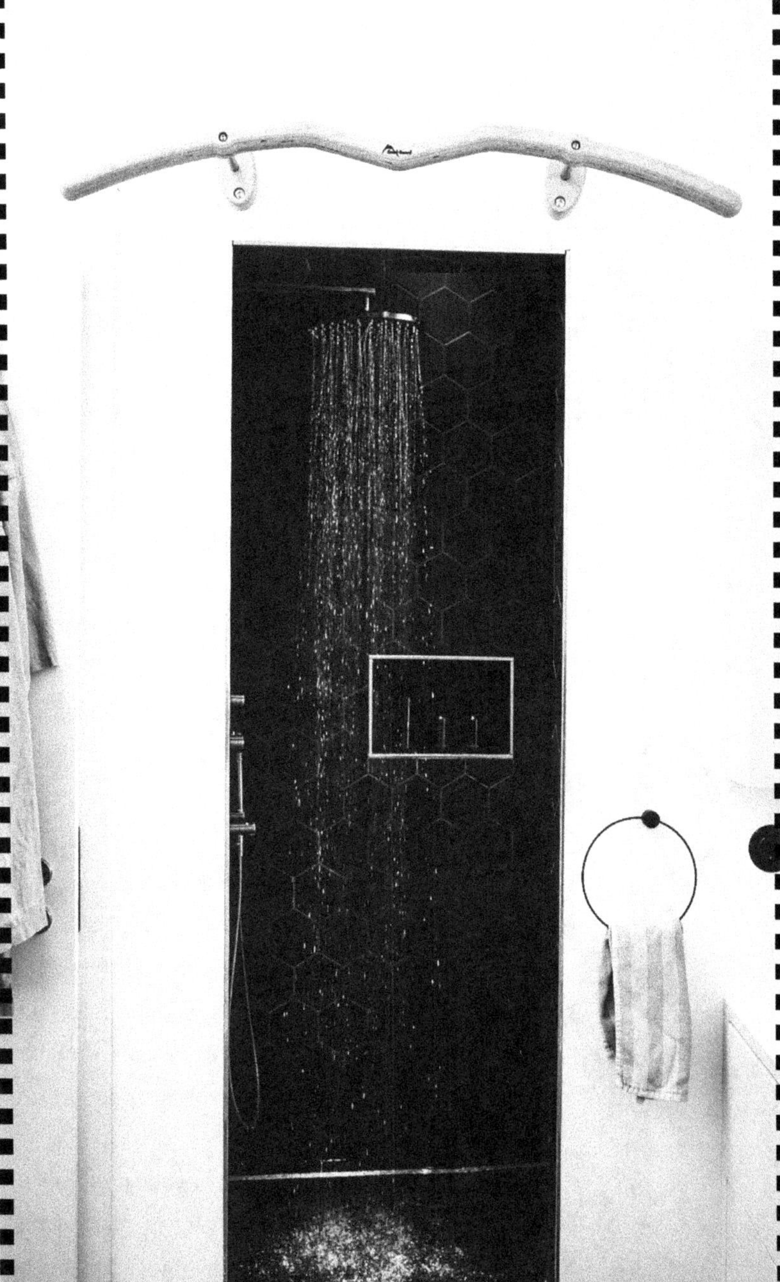

LET YOUR TOOTHBRUSH BE YOUR COACH

Do you sometimes leave the house in the morning without brushing your teeth? Maybe on Monday because you're still a little groggy from the weekend? Or do you skip it on casual Friday?

Few would notice if you did. Besides, your teeth are hardly going to fall out for one missed brushing. It's not the end of the world, but we won't even for a moment consider skipping a session. The tooth-brushing routine might as well be carved in stone, so firmly ingrained is this ritual in our lives. And that is exactly what your daily training has to become—a ritual. You can recognize a ritual by the fact that you don't have to think about *whether* or *how* you're going to do it.[19]

The litmus test for a ritual looks something like this: Say you wake up late with a hangover on the morning of your best friend's wedding and you're in a mad rush to make it on time. Your workout has become a ritual if you still do your push-ups before showering without pausing to give it a second thought.

If thoughts of "not today" cross your mind even for a fleeting moment, your fitness plan is on shaky ground. Economist Clayton Christensen has a 100-percent rule for situations like this.[20] He postulates that it's easier to stick to your principles 100 percent of the time than stay with the program 98 percent of the time.

You've lost the moment you start making room for gray areas and allowing for exceptions. That sounds harsh, but it gets to the crux of the matter.

The going gets a lot easier if you ride in the slipstream of another habit. Let your brushing routine be that vehicle. Knock your 60 seconds of training out as soon you set your toothbrush aside. That has become the morning ritual for my magic minute of training. The toothbrush is my coach. When I put it down, it's time to start training.

If you're thinking about the right time for your workout, I recommend first thing in the morning. Exercise gets your heart pumping, your muscles going and oxygen into your bloodstream. What better way to kick-start your morning? It's your first little victory of the day and a point of pride that puts a bounce in your step: *Exercise? I've already done some today.* I like the way that feels, which is another reason why on every training day I will not step into the shower until after I have done one minute of chin-ups or push-ups. By every day, I don't mean sometimes or often. **I mean always, 100 percent every day.**

THE BEST WAY TO KICK-START YOUR MORNING

THE WORKOUT

CHIN-UPS

Many people can't manage a chin-up, so they have a lot of respect for the exercise. Some consider the chin-up to be the king of upper body exercises because you literally have to pull your own weight. On the following pages, I will show you how to get started with chin-ups. Let me assure you, you will be able to do them regardless of what you happen to weigh. With the right approach, there is no such thing as too hard.

First I'm going to show you how to take some or even a lot of your bodyweight out of the equation. Then we'll break the chin-up down into small, easy-to-do steps. Even if you can't complete a full chin-up just yet, half a chin-up or even just a quarter or fifth of one can get your training off to a good start. The important thing is to push—or in this case, pull—yourself to the limit, to the point where you can't do one more repetition. This is how you strengthen your muscles as described in CHAPTER 5. Do this, and it will only be matter of time before you complete your first full chin-up.

SMALL EASY STEPS

Special rubber bands are available so you don't have to pull your whole bodyweight. Many vendors sell them. You'll get lots of hits if you search the internet for pull-up band or pull-up assist band. When shopping for a band, be sure to consider its weight resistance, which is usually given in pounds or kilograms. This figure tells how much of your weight the band will bear.

LET'S NOT GET AHEAD OF OURSELVES

Simply strap the band to the chin-up bar to lighten your load. Then you can work with less than your full bodyweight, say, to pull up just half your weight. The weight reduction depends on the band's strength. Start with a stronger band and gradually increase the training effect by switching to weaker and weaker bands until you no longer need any assistance. But let's not get ahead of ourselves.

If, like most people, you can't do a chin-up, you should start with a band that can support about half your bodyweight. If you can do one or two chin-ups, go with a band that can bear around one third of your bodyweight. The weight resistance of the left band pictured here is around 35 kilograms (77 pounds) compared to just 12 kilograms (26 pounds) for the narrower one on the right. The wider the band, the more weight it will generally bear.

Once you've found the best
band for your needs,

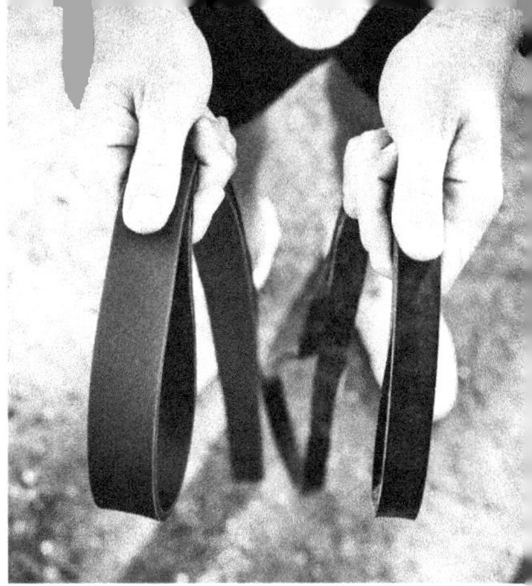

drape it over your chin-up bar as
shown, pulling one loop through
the other.

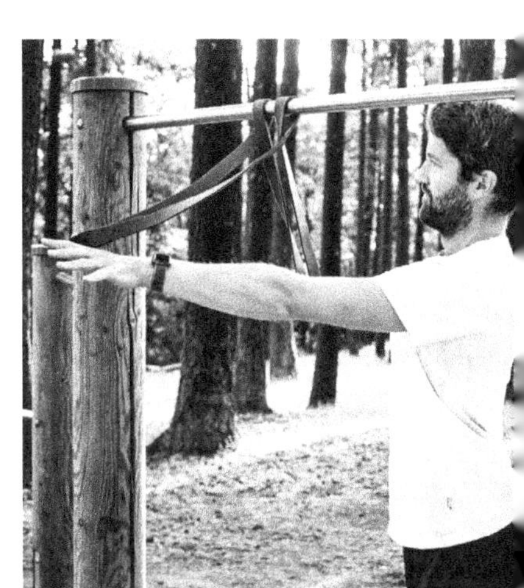

Then pull the loop tight around
the bar.

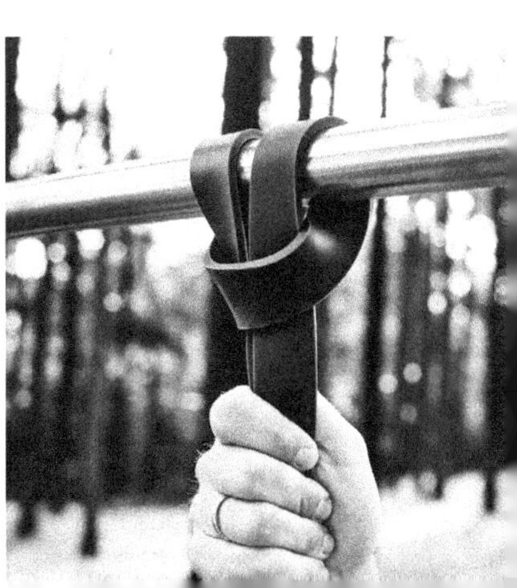

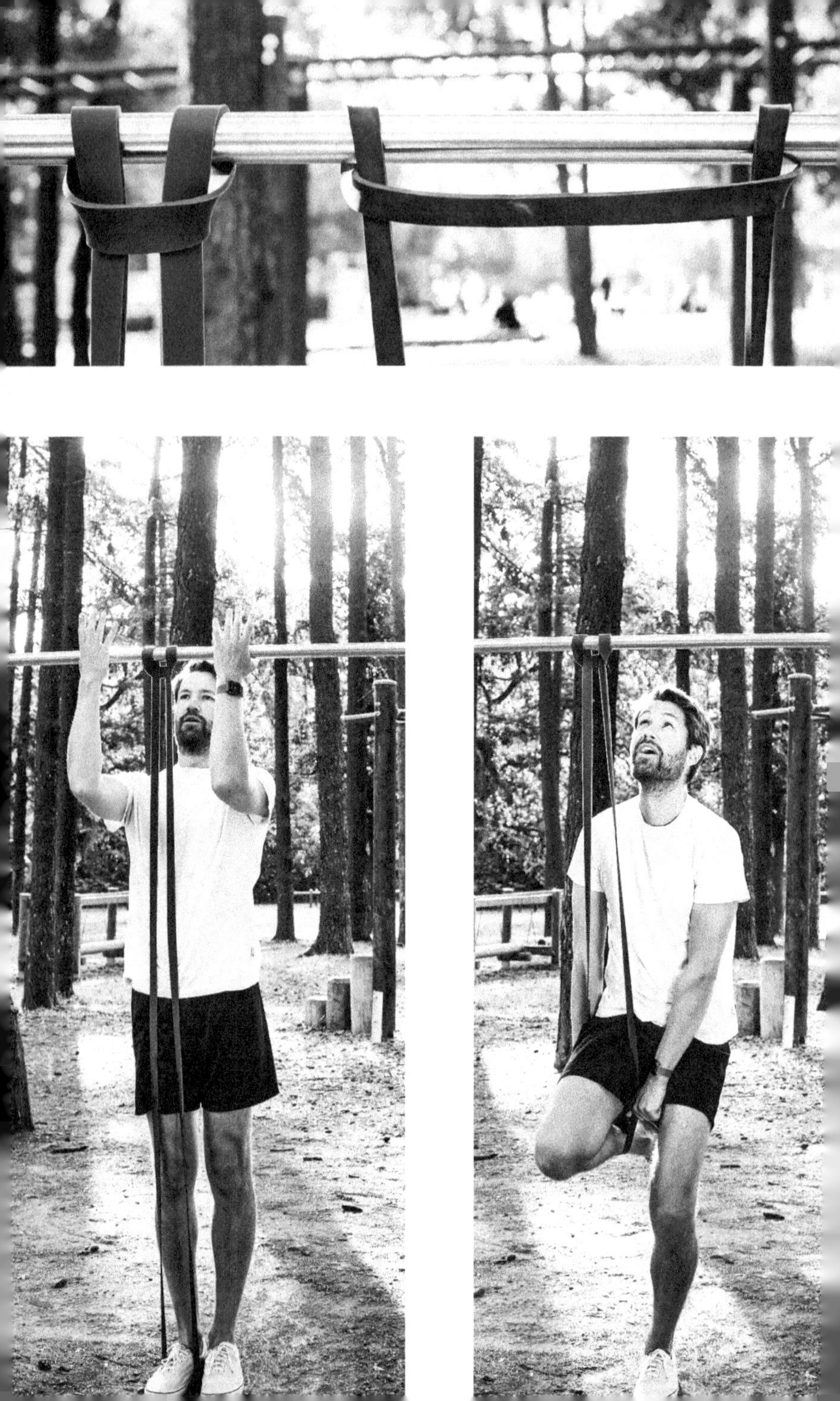

If you need more assistance, widen the loop around the bar so your band looks like the one on the right in the image below. This shortens the load-carrying length of the band to increase resistance so it pulls more of your bodyweight.

You can also vary the amount of support the band provides by placing a foot or a knee in the loop. For maximum support, step into the band with one foot and then push it down to the floor.

You'll get a little less tension and therefore less support for your chin-ups if you thread a knee into the loop. Another advantage of this option is that you don't have to be quite as flexible as you do when stepping high to reach the loop with your foot. Knee or foot, the decision is up to you.

FOR MAXIMUM SUPPORT

You can increase the intensity of your training over the course of weeks and months by using increasingly narrower and weaker bands. Once you can train for a full minute with one band, step down to the next weaker one, and eventually down to none at all. This way, you continue to use your minute efficiently by working out with the intensity and progressive resistance that the science tells us will work.

REPETITIONS

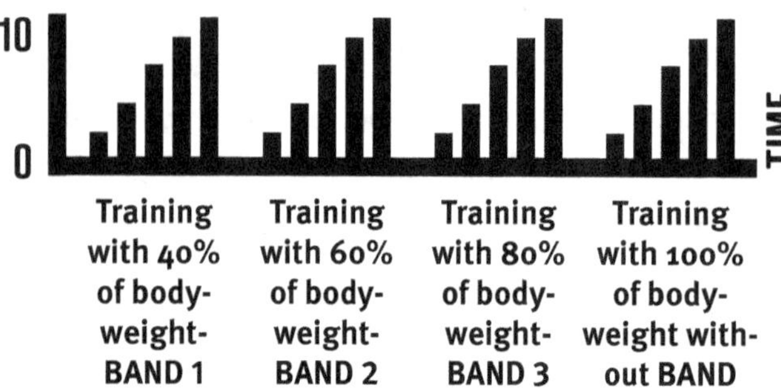

Now you're ready to go for your first half chin-up. The most important thing in performing the chin-up is to do it correctly, with proper form. Never forget the golden rule: *It's better to do a few chin-ups the right way than lots of them the wrong way*. Over time, clean chin-ups done with proper form will build up the muscles that strengthen your back. Sloppy chin-ups can actually harm your back.

So let's go through the exercise step by step:

The starting stance

Before each chin-up, take a moment to get into the correct starting stance. Stand upright at the bar and raise your chest toward it slightly, causing your shoulder blades to move toward each other. Keep your eyes straight ahead and make sure your spine is as straight as possible, particularly the cervical spine or neck region. This little preparatory routine will do two things for you: First, it helps you focus so you concentrate on nothing but the exercise and its proper execution. You only have a minute, so you have to make every movement count by doing it correctly.

Second, your posture will tell you if you are doing the exercise properly. If your head and spine remain locked in place throughout the exercise, maintaining the same posture you started with, then you're doing it right. By that I mean

- head straight
- chest forward
- shoulder blades in
- shoulders down below the base of the neck

Concentrate on holding this posture throughout the workout.

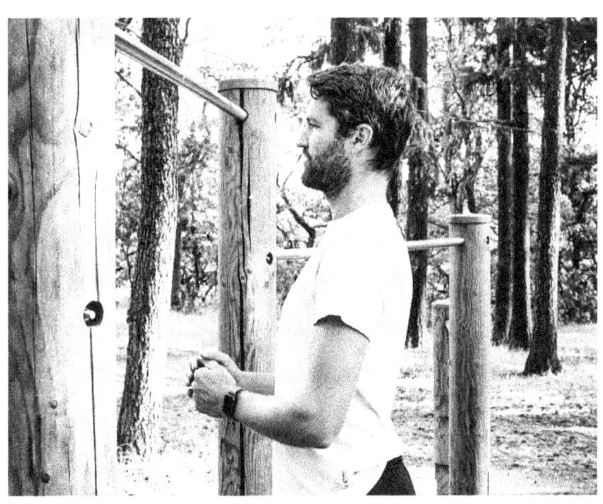

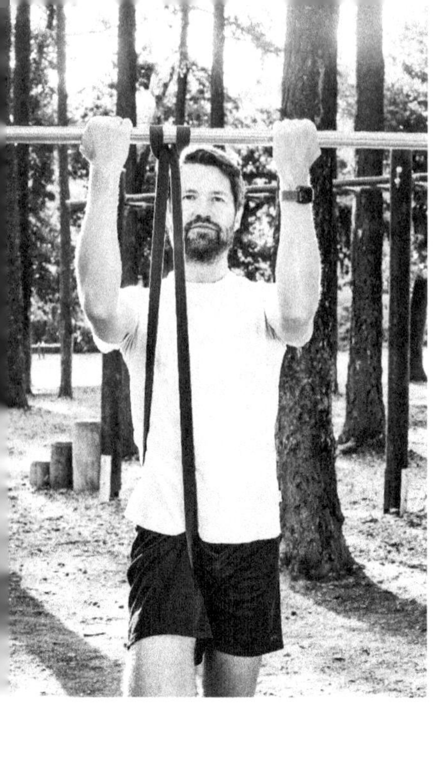
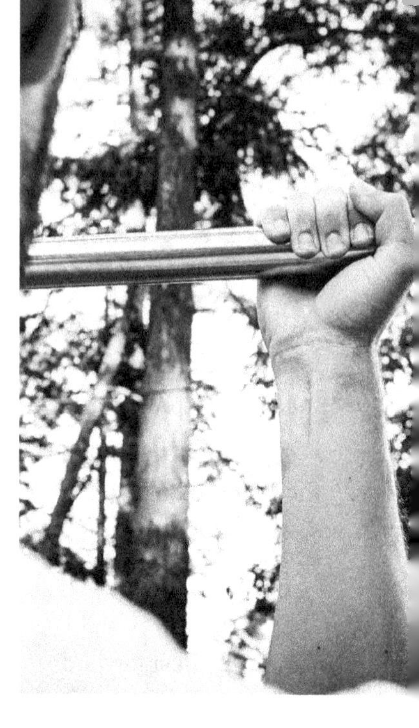
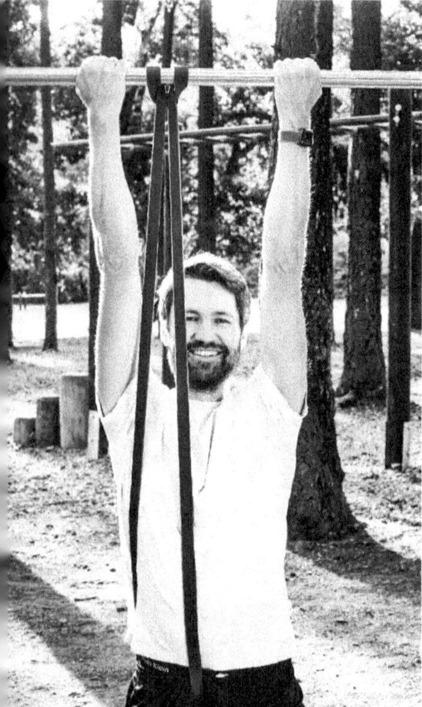
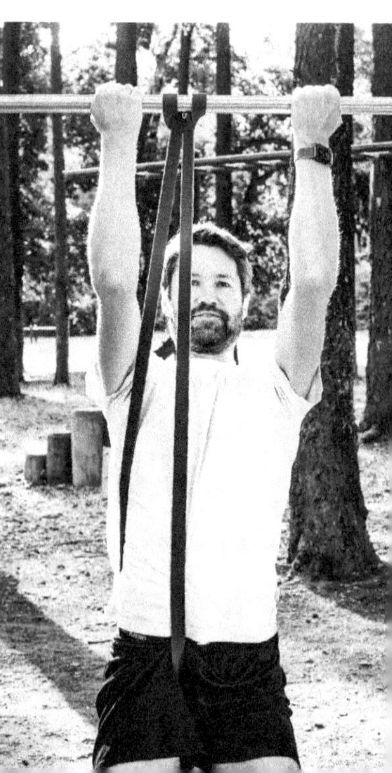

Getting a grip

Grab the bar, placing your hands shoulder-width apart with your palms facing toward you. This is called a pronated or underhand grip. Park your thumbs on your index fingers. This is their natural gripping position, so it should not cause discomfort.

Going down

You want to end up hanging from the bar with your arms fully extended and your elbows straight. Make sure you lower your body very slowly into a dead hang. The downward or negative movement should take around three full seconds. Go all the way down until your arms are fully extended and your elbows straight. Do not let gravity do all the work. Put some muscle into it, applying enough strength to lower your body in a controlled movement. Once your elbows are fully extended, hold the bottom position for a full second, keeping your muscles tensed. This is important, particularly to avoid overstraining your shoulders.

Going up

The first 10 to 20 centimeters (4 to 8 inches) of the ascending or positive movement are very important. This initial leg of your upward journey sets the course for proper execution with a full range of motion. Concentrate on pulling your elbows down.
You're doing it right when your forearms are at right

angles to the bar. You will automatically feel your shoulder blades moving toward each other.

You may not be strong enough to pull your body up any further when you're just starting this program. When you reach your limit, simply begin your slow, controlled descent as described above. Do not try to force yourself up over the bar if you don't have the strength to do so with proper form. If you push beyond muscle failure, your form will get sloppy and all the health benefits of this exercise will go out the window.

SORE ENOUGH TOMORROW

If you have enough strength to continue your ascent, keep pulling your elbows further down until they point straight toward the ground and your chin is up above the bar.

When you reach the highest point, take a moment to make sure your head and shoulders are in the proper position and your posture is still correct. Your elbows are pointing down, eyes are looking straight ahead, neck is straight, shoulder blades are working toward your spine and your chest is moving toward the chin-up bar.

Also make sure that your shoulders remain below the base of your neck.

This is where we're particularly prone to making mistakes. You may be tempted to bring your shoulders up and tuck your neck in to recruit every muscle you have to help you complete your ascent. Please don't

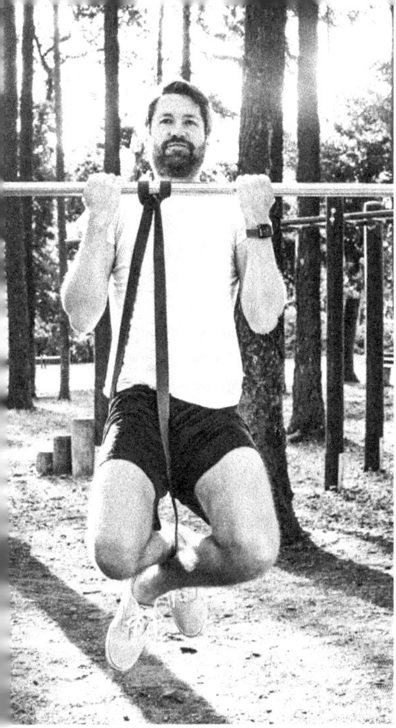

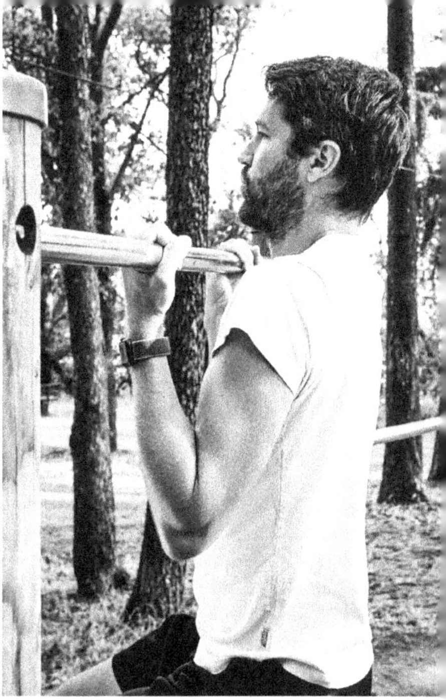

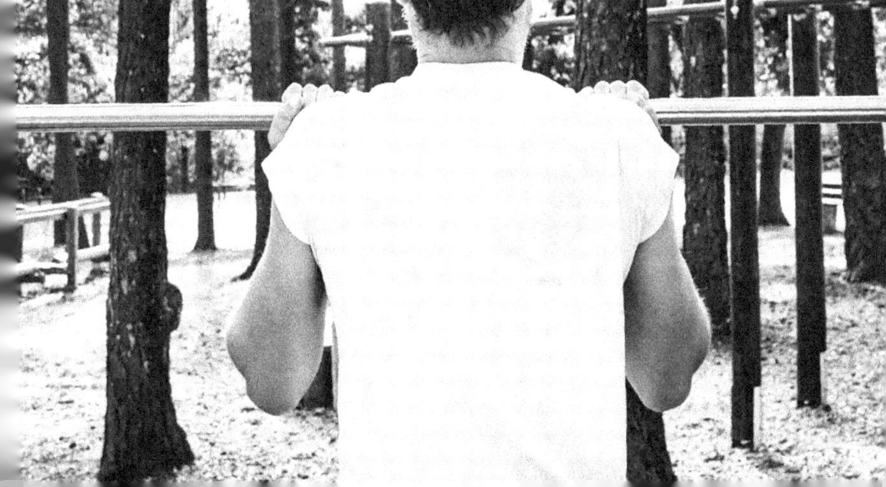

do that! The moment you feel you lack the strength to continue your ascent, simply begin to descend slowly, in a controlled manner. I assure you, your muscles will still get a proper workout. They'll feel sore enough tomorrow, but you will slowly but surely improve over the weeks and months until you complete your first full chin-up—cleanly, with proper form.

In contrast to the slow descent, your ascent needs to be a fast, dynamic movement that takes you no more than two seconds. Of course, if your bar is high enough that you have to stretch a little to grab it, you're already at the bottom position. Start your ascent from there. Otherwise, the procedure is the same as above.

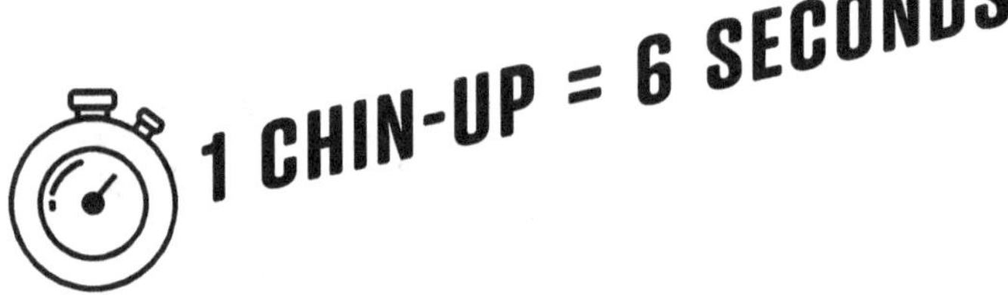

A complete and cleanly executed chin-up takes about six seconds:

- lower your body for three seconds
- at the lowest point, remain at a dead hang for one second
- pull up for two seconds

Your goal is push yourself to the limit by completing ten chin-ups with proper form in 60 seconds. It will likely take you weeks or even months to get there. This is completely normal, and everyone progresses at different speeds. **But no matter how many chin-ups you end up doing and regardless of what kind of assistance you use in your training, you always have to push yourself to your limit within 60 seconds.**

Variants

Once you manage to knock out clean chin-ups for 60 seconds without resistance bands to assist you, you will have to increase the training stimulus to achieve further progress. There are many variants of the chin-up that can increase the intensity of your one-minute workout. As a fringe benefit, they work the muscle groups in different ways for an added training effect, so it also makes sense to integrate these variants into your routine at an early stage.

First, I recommend that you try a supinated, or overhand, grip to perform pull-ups. Bands can assist you with this variant, as well. Keeping your hands shoulder-width apart, grab the bar with your palms facing away from your body, toward the bar. The pull-up is a more demanding ex-

INCREASE THE TRAINING STIMULUS

ercise as your arms do less of the work. Another way of increasing the training stimulus is to vary the grip width. The overhand grip lets you place your hands closer together or farther apart than shoulder width. The underhand grip does not lend itself to a very wide grip. Your wrists will be the first to protest if you try that. As you begin to make progress with your training, I recommend you start varying the type and width of your grip. **For the basic level of fitness we want to achieve with the daily 60-second routine, you don't need to increase the intensity beyond that.**

VARY THE GRIP WIDTH

PUSH-UPS

You may recall from CHAPTER 3 that the push-up is the perfect complement to the chin-up. The chin-up trains the flexors and the push-up takes care of the extenders. The push-up is also somewhat easier to perform than the chin-up. However, that that is precisely why it demands concentration on your part. When we think of something being easy, our focus tends to drift. If we do that with the push-up, we will end up executing the exercise incorrectly or haphazardly. So let's look at how to do a push-up properly.

Getting set

Get down on all fours, placing your hands on the floor directly below your shoulders and about shoulder-width apart. Extend one foot back and then the other, raising up on bent toes. Keep your feet close together to fix your heels in place and stabilize your position during the exercise. Make sure that your shoulders, glutes and heels form a straight line. Beginners tend to instinctively bend at the hip to relieve the core muscles. If necessary, have your partner or a friend correct your stance. Keep your back straight and neutral; don't arch it by allowing your hips to dip toward the floor or rise toward the

KEEP BACK STRAIGHT AND NEUTRAL

ceiling. If you do all this properly, you will automatically engage your abdominal muscles. It you feel them tense up, you're on your way to getting your posture right.

The starting position is as important to the push-up as it is to the chin-up. Before doing your first push up, always take a moment to check whether your posture is correct. Once you've done that, take a second to compose yourself and focus, then off you go.

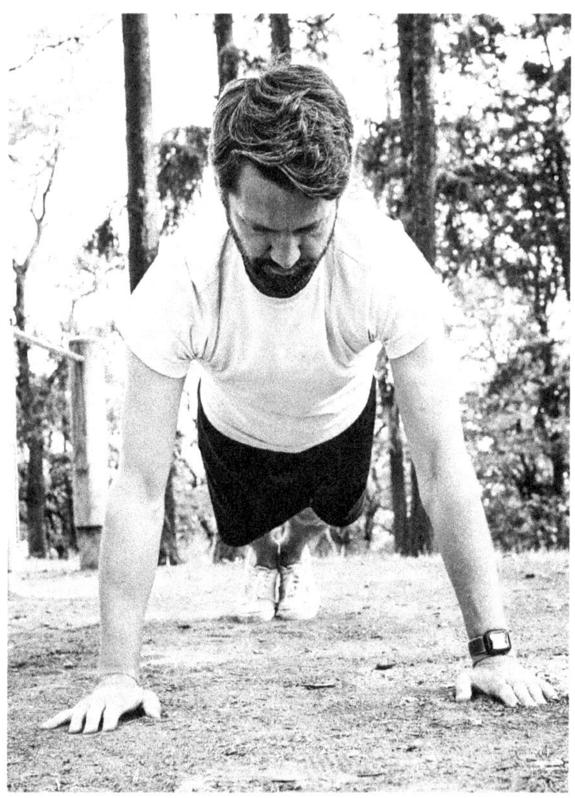

Going down

The downward motion starts at the elbows. Bend them back toward your feet. This is the most important initial movement. You will feel your shoulder blades move toward each other, not unlike they do for a chin-up. Keep the position of your shoulder blades in mind throughout the exercise. The big mistakes come at the start, with the elbows moving out to the sides to take the load off the shoulders. If you allow that to happen, the exercise will be inefficient and much of your effort will be in vain!

KEEP YOUR SHOULDER BLADES IN MIND

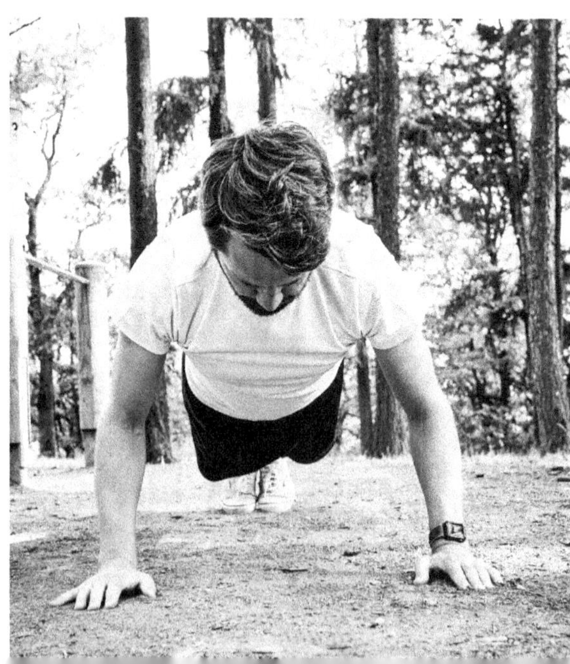

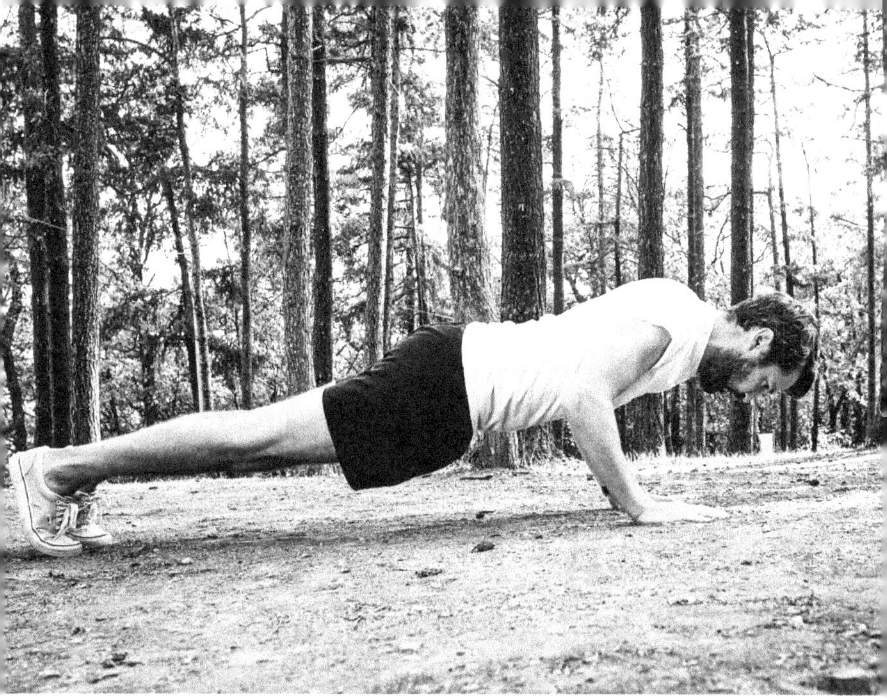

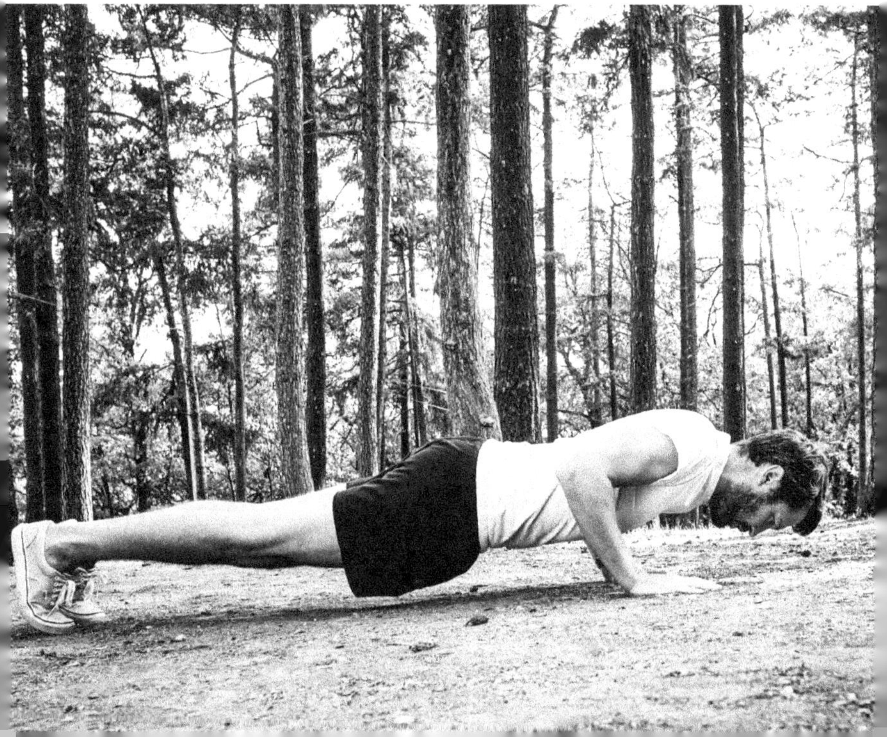

Keeping your shoulders, back, glutes and feet in a straight line is essential during the first few centimeters on your way down. If you hold that line, you will feel the muscle tension from head to toe.

MUSCLE TENSION FROM HEAD TO TOE

Your shoulder, abdominal and gluteal muscles are all engaged, as are your thighs and calves. Get used to feeling these tensed muscles—this will help you maintain proper form. If you lose this tension because you've relaxed a certain muscle, then it's likely your line—which is so important to the exercise's effectiveness—will no longer be straight.

Hold that line as you lower your body until the tip of your nose touches the ground. This movement should keep you busy for about two seconds.

If you did everything right on the way down, your elbows will be tucked in very close to your upper body. Stay in this position, maintaining full muscle tension for one second. Then focus on pushing your body up in a straight line.

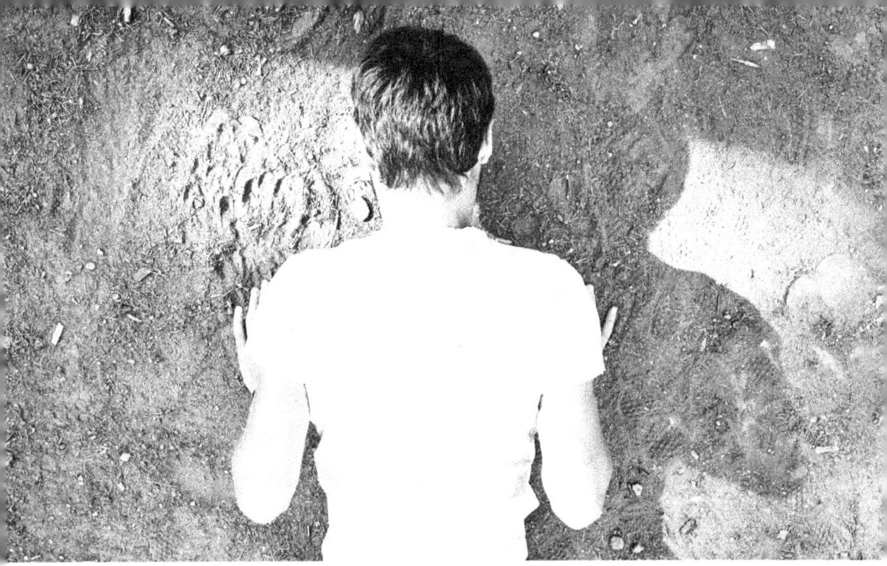

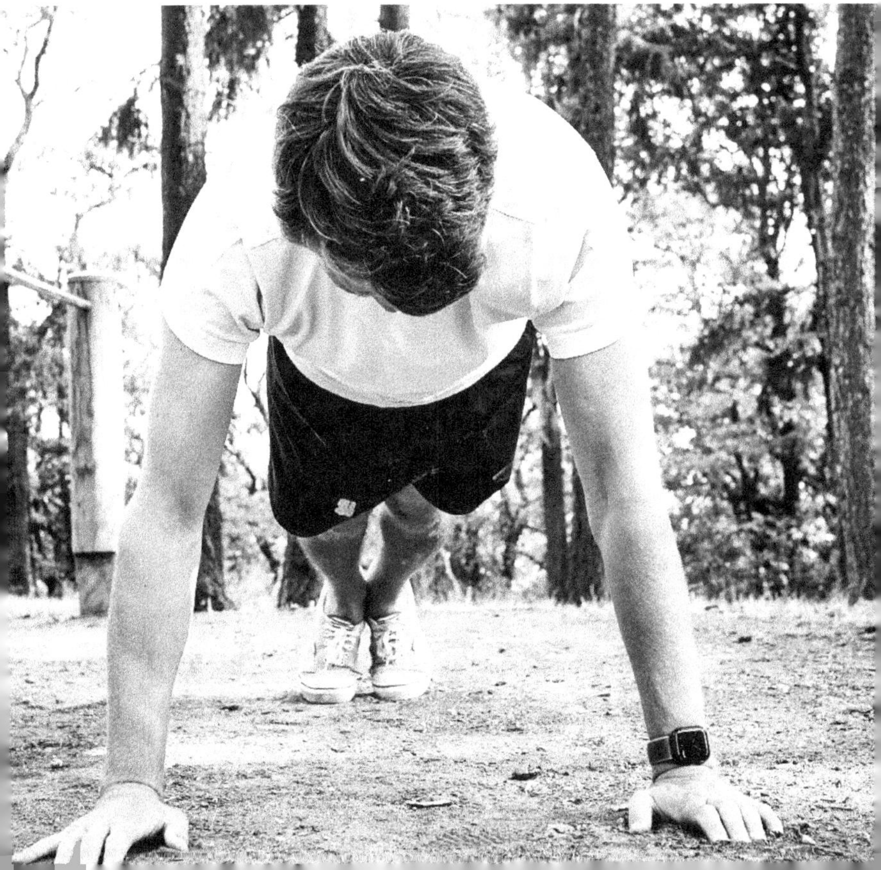

Pushing up

To return to the up position, follow the same procedure that brought you down, but in reverse order. Remember, it is important to keep your elbows in close to your upper body.

If you do this, you will feel your shoulders engaging again to take up some of the load. Be sure to hold your shoulder blades in that position to keep the muscle tension constant.

Now push yourself up until your elbows are extended. One second should be enough time to go from the down to the up position. You do not need to pause

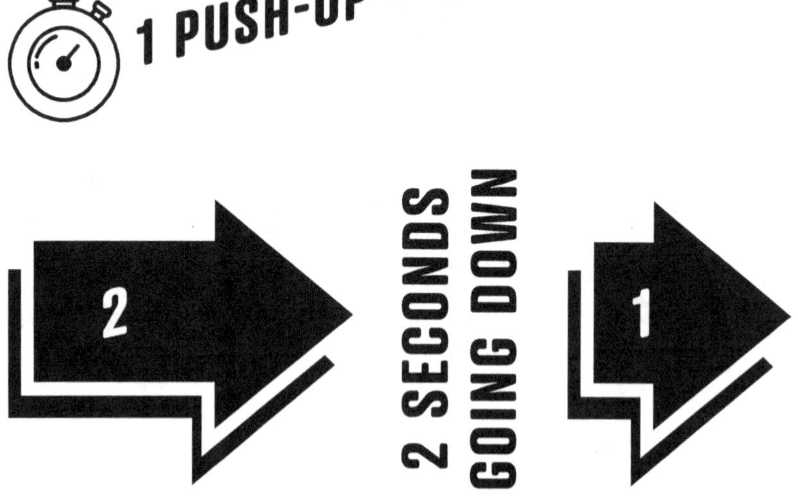

when you reach the top. As soon as you have fully extended your arms, immediately begin lowering your body again. It should take you around four seconds to complete a full push-up:

- descend for two seconds
- hold for one second at the lowest point
- push up in one second

enabling you to complete 15 repetitions in one minute.

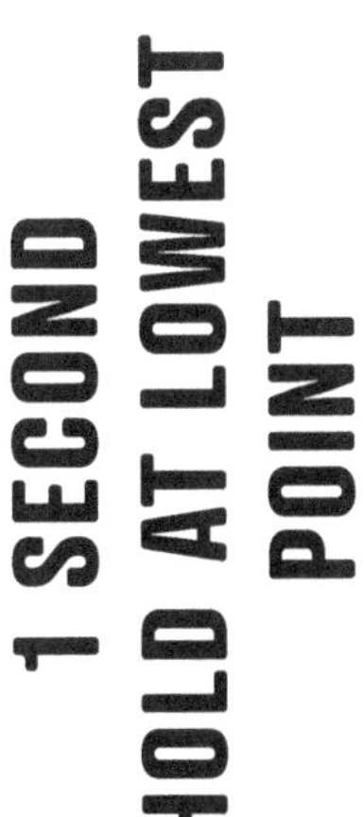

Variants

What we said for the chin-up holds true for the push up as well: you will have to mix it up once you reach the point where the standard exercise no longer pushes you to your limit. You have various options, the easiest being to change the position of your hands. In the standard version, they are around shoulder-width apart. You can move them closer together or further apart to change the load and stimulate your muscles in different ways. You can also try push-up bars or handles. They extend your range of motion, which makes the exercise harder for your muscles, but easier on your wrists. Once you have mastered that added level of difficulty, you can step up to the ultimate challenge of the one-arm push-up.

THE ULTIMATE CHALLENGE

Let's go

You now have everything you need to start building your foundation for physical fitness—a sense of urgency, low entry barriers, the *mover matrix*, two old but gold exercises rediscovered, and a previously undiscovered purpose for your toothbrush...

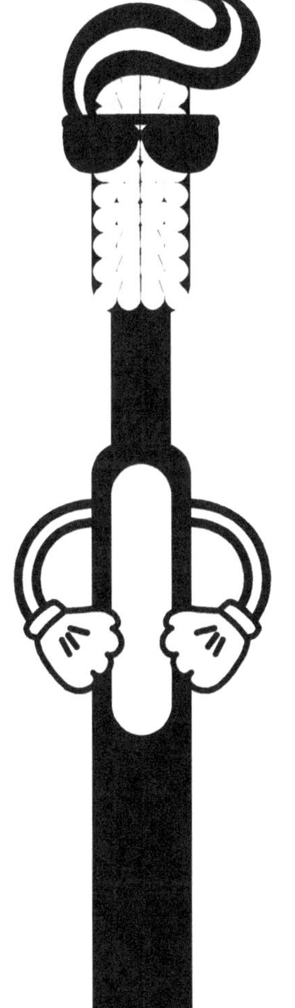

ACKNOWLEDGEMENTS

The approach described in this book is effective, as the story of how it came about attests. The idea for FIT IN NO TIME had been on my mind for five long years. Inspired by the Canadian study that examined the viability of a one-minute workout, I had a program together to train my—at the time woefully weak—back within a few days. Finding the right twin-pack of exercises was easy with the help of my rock-climbing friend. The challenge of toning it down for beginners was tackled in the space of a few evenings and various experiments with climbing harnesses, pulleys and resistance bands. I invented the *mover matrix* on my way to work, my boss at the time being a big fan of decision matrices. And I came across the 100-percent rule in an article I had read while brushing my teeth. All the parts were in place in less than six weeks.

My attempts to write the book were less auspicious. I found that I *simply did not have enough time for it,* an observation that has become all too familiar to me. For five years, I tried and failed to find space in my busy life for this book. Then one day its premise prompted in me the right question: *How do I write a book in one minute a day?*

The answer was teamwork. I would not have been able to do it alone—certainly not with the resources left after living up to family and work commitments. This is why my heartfelt gratitude goes out to the wonderful team that made this book possible—to Laura Schöffel for her help with the text and debates about content, to Lisa Beller and Lasse Schneider for the pictures taken in the sunshine, to Konstantin Hauck for invaluable ideas about time and structure, to Michelle Sattinger for a wonderful editing job, and to the team at Schönski Design Studio for all the eye candy that makes this a fun read.

The *mover matrix* may well be the most valuable exercise in this book. If you become aware of your goals and match them up with the resources you really have available, you will find creative ways to rise to challenges that have long been dogging your footsteps—**perhaps even longer than the five years that this book hounded me.**

YOUR TRAINING JOURNAL

FIT IN NO TIME consists of just two exercises, but that doesn't diminish the importance of tracking your progress. You need to do this to train effectively. Besides, seeing your goals achieved is sweet satisfaction indeed. I've included a journal you can use to track your training performance and progress. **Take it from one who knows: you will appreciate that log when you find yourself struggling to answer the question that keeps coming up every morning—is today chin-up or push-up day?**

WEEK 1   from   to

MON	TUE	WED	THU	FRI	SAT	SD
Chin-ups	Push-ups	Chin-ups	Push-ups	Chin-ups	Push-ups	REST
Repe-titions	Repe-titions	Repe-titions	Repe-titions	Repe-titions	Repe-titions	
Overhand ☐ Underhand ☐ Shoulder-width ☐ Wider ☐ Band-strength	Push-Up-Bars ☐ One arm ☐ Shoulder-width ☐	Overhand ☐ Underhand ☐ Shoulder-width ☐ Wider ☐ Band-strength	Push-Up-Bars ☐ One arm ☐ Shoulder-width ☐	Overhand ☐ Underhand ☐ Shoulder-width ☐ Wider ☐ Band-strength	Push-Up-Bars ☐ One arm ☐ Shoulder-width ☐	

WEEK 2   from   to

MON	TUE	WED	THU	FRI	SAT	SD
Chin-ups	Push-ups	Chin-ups	Push-ups	Chin-ups	Push-ups	REST
Repe-titions	Repe-titions	Repe-titions	Repe-titions	Repe-titions	Repe-titions	
Overhand ☐ Underhand ☐ Shoulder-width ☐ Wider ☐ Band-strength	Push-Up-Bars ☐ One arm ☐ Shoulder-width ☐	Overhand ☐ Underhand ☐ Shoulder-width ☐ Wider ☐ Band-strength	Push-Up-Bars ☐ One arm ☐ Shoulder-width ☐	Overhand ☐ Underhand ☐ Shoulder-width ☐ Wider ☐ Band-strength	Push-Up-Bars ☐ One arm ☐ Shoulder-width ☐	

WEEK 3   from   to

MON	TUE	WED	THU	FRI	SAT	SD
Chin-ups	**Push-ups**	**Chin-ups**	**Push-ups**	**Chin-ups**	**Push-ups**	REST
Repe-titions	Repe-titions	Repe-titions	Repe-titions	Repe-titions	Repe-titions	
Overhand ☐ Underhand ☐ Shoulder-width ☐ Wider ☐ Band-strength	Push-Up-Bars ☐ One arm ☐ Shoulder-width ☐	Overhand ☐ Underhand ☐ Shoulder-width ☐ Wider ☐ Band-strength	Push-Up-Bars ☐ One arm ☐ Shoulder-width ☐	Overhand ☐ Underhand ☐ Shoulder-width ☐ Wider ☐ Band-strength	Push-Up-Bars ☐ One arm ☐ Shoulder-width ☐	

WEEK 4   from   to

MON	TUE	WED	THU	FRI	SAT	SD
Chin-ups	**Push-ups**	**Chin-ups**	**Push-ups**	**Chin-ups**	**Push-ups**	REST
Repe-titions	Repe-titions	Repe-titions	Repe-titions	Repe-titions	Repe-titions	
Overhand ☐ Underhand ☐ Shoulder-width ☐ Wider ☐ Band-strength	Push-Up-Bars ☐ One arm ☐ Shoulder-width ☐	Overhand ☐ Underhand ☐ Shoulder-width ☐ Wider ☐ Band-strength	Push-Up-Bars ☐ One arm ☐ Shoulder-width ☐	Overhand ☐ Underhand ☐ Shoulder-width ☐ Wider ☐ Band-strength	Push-Up-Bars ☐ One arm ☐ Shoulder-width ☐	

WEEK 5   from   to

MON	TUE	WED	THU	FRI	SAT	SD
Chin-ups	**Push-ups**	**Chin-ups**	**Push-ups**	**Chin-ups**	**Push-ups**	
Repe-titions	Repe-titions	Repe-titions	Repe-titions	Repe-titions	Repe-titions	
Overhand ☐ Underhand ☐ Shoulder-width ☐ Wider ☐ Band-strength	Push-Up-Bars ☐ One arm ☐ Shoulder-width ☐	Overhand ☐ Underhand ☐ Shoulder-width ☐ Wider ☐ Band-strength	Push-Up-Bars ☐ One arm ☐ Shoulder-width ☐	Overhand ☐ Underhand ☐ Shoulder-width ☐ Wider ☐ Band-strength	Push-Up-Bars ☐ One arm ☐ Shoulder-width ☐	REST

WEEK 6   from   to

MON	TUE	WED	THU	FRI	SAT	SD
Chin-ups	**Push-ups**	**Chin-ups**	**Push-ups**	**Chin-ups**	**Push-ups**	
Repe-titions	Repe-titions	Repe-titions	Repe-titions	Repe-titions	Repe-titions	
Overhand ☐ Underhand ☐ Shoulder-width ☐ Wider ☐ Band-strength	Push-Up-Bars ☐ One arm ☐ Shoulder-width ☐	Overhand ☐ Underhand ☐ Shoulder-width ☐ Wider ☐ Band-strength	Push-Up-Bars ☐ One arm ☐ Shoulder-width ☐	Overhand ☐ Underhand ☐ Shoulder-width ☐ Wider ☐ Band-strength	Push-Up-Bars ☐ One arm ☐ Shoulder-width ☐	REST

WEEK 7   from   to

MON	TUE	WED	THU	FRI	SAT	SD
Chin-ups	**Push-ups**	**Chin-ups**	**Push-ups**	**Chin-ups**	**Push-ups**	
Repe-titions	Repe-titions	Repe-titions	Repe-titions	Repe-titions	Repe-titions	
Overhand ☐ Underhand ☐ Shoulder-width ☐ Wider ☐ Band-strength	Push-Up-Bars ☐ One arm ☐ Shoulder-width ☐	Overhand ☐ Underhand ☐ Shoulder-width ☐ Wider ☐ Band-strength	Push-Up-Bars ☐ One arm ☐ Shoulder-width ☐	Overhand ☐ Underhand ☐ Shoulder-width ☐ Wider ☐ Band-strength	Push-Up-Bars ☐ One arm ☐ Shoulder-width ☐	REST

WEEK 8   from   to

MON	TUE	WED	THU	FRI	SAT	SD
Chin-ups	**Push-ups**	**Chin-ups**	**Push-ups**	**Chin-ups**	**Push-ups**	
Repe-titions	Repe-titions	Repe-titions	Repe-titions	Repe-titions	Repe-titions	
Overhand ☐ Underhand ☐ Shoulder-width ☐ Wider ☐ Band-strength	Push-Up-Bars ☐ One arm ☐ Shoulder-width ☐	Overhand ☐ Underhand ☐ Shoulder-width ☐ Wider ☐ Band-strength	Push-Up-Bars ☐ One arm ☐ Shoulder-width ☐	Overhand ☐ Underhand ☐ Shoulder-width ☐ Wider ☐ Band-strength	Push-Up-Bars ☐ One arm ☐ Shoulder-width ☐	REST

WEEK 9

from　　　　　　to

MON	TUE	WED	THU	FRI	SAT	SD
Chin-ups	**Push-ups**	**Chin-ups**	**Push-ups**	**Chin-ups**	**Push-ups**	REST
Repetitions	Repetitions	Repetitions	Repetitions	Repetitions	Repetitions	
Overhand ☐ Underhand ☐ Shoulder-width ☐ Wider ☐ Band-strength	Push-Up-Bars ☐ One arm ☐ Shoulder-width ☐	Overhand ☐ Underhand ☐ Shoulder-width ☐ Wider ☐ Band-strength	Push-Up-Bars ☐ One arm ☐ Shoulder-width ☐	Overhand ☐ Underhand ☐ Shoulder-width ☐ Wider ☐ Band-strength	Push-Up-Bars ☐ One arm ☐ Shoulder-width ☐	

WEEK 10

from　　　　　　to

MON	TUE	WED	THU	FRI	SAT	SD
Chin-ups	**Push-ups**	**Chin-ups**	**Push-ups**	**Chin-ups**	**Push-ups**	REST
Repetitions	Repetitions	Repetitions	Repetitions	Repetitions	Repetitions	
Overhand ☐ Underhand ☐ Shoulder-width ☐ Wider ☐ Band-strength	Push-Up-Bars ☐ One arm ☐ Shoulder-width ☐	Overhand ☐ Underhand ☐ Shoulder-width ☐ Wider ☐ Band-strength	Push-Up-Bars ☐ One arm ☐ Shoulder-width ☐	Overhand ☐ Underhand ☐ Shoulder-width ☐ Wider ☐ Band-strength	Push-Up-Bars ☐ One arm ☐ Shoulder-width ☐	

WEEK 11   from   to

MON	TUE	WED	THU	FRI	SAT	SD
Chin-ups	**Push-ups**	**Chin-ups**	**Push-ups**	**Chin-ups**	**Push-ups**	
Repetitions	Repetitions	Repetitions	Repetitions	Repetitions	Repetitions	
Overhand ☐ Underhand ☐ Shoulder-width ☐ Wider ☐ Band-strength	Push-Up-Bars ☐ One arm ☐ Shoulder-width ☐	Overhand ☐ Underhand ☐ Shoulder-width ☐ Wider ☐ Band-strength	Push-Up-Bars ☐ One arm ☐ Shoulder-width ☐	Overhand ☐ Underhand ☐ Shoulder-width ☐ Wider ☐ Band-strength	Push-Up-Bars ☐ One arm ☐ Shoulder-width ☐	REST

WEEK 12   from   to

MON	TUE	WED	THU	FRI	SAT	SD
Chin-ups	**Push-ups**	**Chin-ups**	**Push-ups**	**Chin-ups**	**Push-ups**	
Repetitions	Repetitions	Repetitions	Repetitions	Repetitions	Repetitions	
Overhand ☐ Underhand ☐ Shoulder-width ☐ Wider ☐ Band-strength	Push-Up-Bars ☐ One arm ☐ Shoulder-width ☐	Overhand ☐ Underhand ☐ Shoulder-width ☐ Wider ☐ Band-strength	Push-Up-Bars ☐ One arm ☐ Shoulder-width ☐	Overhand ☐ Underhand ☐ Shoulder-width ☐ Wider ☐ Band-strength	Push-Up-Bars ☐ One arm ☐ Shoulder-width ☐	REST

WEEK 13   from   to

MON	TUE	WED	THU	FRI	SAT	SD
Chin-ups	**Push-ups**	**Chin-ups**	**Push-ups**	**Chin-ups**	**Push-ups**	
Repe-titions	Repe-titions	Repe-titions	Repe-titions	Repe-titions	Repe-titions	
Overhand ☐ Underhand ☐ Shoulder-width ☐ Wider ☐ Band-strength	Push-Up-Bars ☐ One arm ☐ Shoulder-width ☐	Overhand ☐ Underhand ☐ Shoulder-width ☐ Wider ☐ Band-strength	Push-Up-Bars ☐ One arm ☐ Shoulder-width ☐	Overhand ☐ Underhand ☐ Shoulder-width ☐ Wider ☐ Band-strength	Push-Up-Bars ☐ One arm ☐ Shoulder-width ☐	REST

WEEK 14   from   to

MON	TUE	WED	THU	FRI	SAT	SD
Chin-ups	**Push-ups**	**Chin-ups**	**Push-ups**	**Chin-ups**	**Push-ups**	
Repe-titions	Repe-titions	Repe-titions	Repe-titions	Repe-titions	Repe-titions	
Overhand ☐ Underhand ☐ Shoulder-width ☐ Wider ☐ Band-strength	Push-Up-Bars ☐ One arm ☐ Shoulder-width ☐	Overhand ☐ Underhand ☐ Shoulder-width ☐ Wider ☐ Band-strength	Push-Up-Bars ☐ One arm ☐ Shoulder-width ☐	Overhand ☐ Underhand ☐ Shoulder-width ☐ Wider ☐ Band-strength	Push-Up-Bars ☐ One arm ☐ Shoulder-width ☐	REST

WEEK 15 from   to

MON	TUE	WED	THU	FRI	SAT	SD
Chin-ups	Push-ups	Chin-ups	Push-ups	Chin-ups	Push-ups	REST
Repetitions	Repetitions	Repetitions	Repetitions	Repetitions	Repetitions	
Overhand ☐ Underhand ☐ Shoulder-width ☐ Wider ☐ Band-strength	Push-Up-Bars ☐ One arm ☐ Shoulder-width ☐	Overhand ☐ Underhand ☐ Shoulder-width ☐ Wider ☐ Band-strength	Push-Up-Bars ☐ One arm ☐ Shoulder-width ☐	Overhand ☐ Underhand ☐ Shoulder-width ☐ Wider ☐ Band-strength	Push-Up-Bars ☐ One arm ☐ Shoulder-width ☐	

WEEK 16 from   to

MON	TUE	WED	THU	FRI	SAT	SD
Chin-ups	Push-ups	Chin-ups	Push-ups	Chin-ups	Push-ups	REST
Repetitions	Repetitions	Repetitions	Repetitions	Repetitions	Repetitions	
Overhand ☐ Underhand ☐ Shoulder-width ☐ Wider ☐ Band-strength	Push-Up-Bars ☐ One arm ☐ Shoulder-width ☐	Overhand ☐ Underhand ☐ Shoulder-width ☐ Wider ☐ Band-strength	Push-Up-Bars ☐ One arm ☐ Shoulder-width ☐	Overhand ☐ Underhand ☐ Shoulder-width ☐ Wider ☐ Band-strength	Push-Up-Bars ☐ One arm ☐ Shoulder-width ☐	

WEEK 17   from   to

MON	TUE	WED	THU	FRI	SAT	SD
Chin-ups	**Push-ups**	**Chin-ups**	**Push-ups**	**Chin-ups**	**Push-ups**	
Repe-titions	Repe-titions	Repe-titions	Repe-titions	Repe-titions	Repe-titions	
Overhand ☐ Underhand ☐ Shoulder-width ☐ Wider ☐ Band-strength	Push-Up-Bars ☐ One arm ☐ Shoulder-width ☐	Overhand ☐ Underhand ☐ Shoulder-width ☐ Wider ☐ Band-strength	Push-Up-Bars ☐ One arm ☐ Shoulder-width ☐	Overhand ☐ Underhand ☐ Shoulder-width ☐ Wider ☐ Band-strength	Push-Up-Bars ☐ One arm ☐ Shoulder-width ☐	REST

WEEK 18   from   to

MON	TUE	WED	THU	FRI	SAT	SD
Chin-ups	**Push-ups**	**Chin-ups**	**Push-ups**	**Chin-ups**	**Push-ups**	
Repe-titions	Repe-titions	Repe-titions	Repe-titions	Repe-titions	Repe-titions	
Overhand ☐ Underhand ☐ Shoulder-width ☐ Wider ☐ Band-strength	Push-Up-Bars ☐ One arm ☐ Shoulder-width ☐	Overhand ☐ Underhand ☐ Shoulder-width ☐ Wider ☐ Band-strength	Push-Up-Bars ☐ One arm ☐ Shoulder-width ☐	Overhand ☐ Underhand ☐ Shoulder-width ☐ Wider ☐ Band-strength	Push-Up-Bars ☐ One arm ☐ Shoulder-width ☐	REST

WEEK 19 from   to

MON	TUE	WED	THU	FRI	SAT	SD
Chin-ups	Push-ups	Chin-ups	Push-ups	Chin-ups	Push-ups	
Repetitions	Repetitions	Repetitions	Repetitions	Repetitions	Repetitions	
Overhand ☐ Underhand ☐ Shoulder-width ☐ Wider ☐ Band-strength	Push-Up-Bars ☐ One arm ☐ Shoulder-width ☐	Overhand ☐ Underhand ☐ Shoulder-width ☐ Wider ☐ Band-strength	Push-Up-Bars ☐ One arm ☐ Shoulder-width ☐	Overhand ☐ Underhand ☐ Shoulder-width ☐ Wider ☐ Band-strength	Push-Up-Bars ☐ One arm ☐ Shoulder-width ☐	REST

WEEK 20 from   to

MON	TUE	WED	THU	FRI	SAT	SD
Chin-ups	Push-ups	Chin-ups	Push-ups	Chin-ups	Push-ups	
Repetitions	Repetitions	Repetitions	Repetitions	Repetitions	Repetitions	
Overhand ☐ Underhand ☐ Shoulder-width ☐ Wider ☐ Band-strength	Push-Up-Bars ☐ One arm ☐ Shoulder-width ☐	Overhand ☐ Underhand ☐ Shoulder-width ☐ Wider ☐ Band-strength	Push-Up-Bars ☐ One arm ☐ Shoulder-width ☐	Overhand ☐ Underhand ☐ Shoulder-width ☐ Wider ☐ Band-strength	Push-Up-Bars ☐ One arm ☐ Shoulder-width ☐	REST

WEEK 21   from   to

MON	TUE	WED	THU	FRI	SAT	SD
Chin-ups	Push-ups	Chin-ups	Push-ups	Chin-ups	Push-ups	REST
Repe-titions	Repe-titions	Repe-titions	Repe-titions	Repe-titions	Repe-titions	
Overhand ☐ Underhand ☐ Shoulder-width ☐ Wider ☐ Band-strength	Push-Up-Bars ☐ One arm ☐ Shoulder-width ☐	Overhand ☐ Underhand ☐ Shoulder-width ☐ Wider ☐ Band-strength	Push-Up-Bars ☐ One arm ☐ Shoulder-width ☐	Overhand ☐ Underhand ☐ Shoulder-width ☐ Wider ☐ Band-strength	Push-Up-Bars ☐ One arm ☐ Shoulder-width ☐	

WEEK 22   from   to

MON	TUE	WED	THU	FRI	SAT	SD
Chin-ups	Push-ups	Chin-ups	Push-ups	Chin-ups	Push-ups	REST
Repe-titions	Repe-titions	Repe-titions	Repe-titions	Repe-titions	Repe-titions	
Overhand ☐ Underhand ☐ Shoulder-width ☐ Wider ☐ Band-strength	Push-Up-Bars ☐ One arm ☐ Shoulder-width ☐	Overhand ☐ Underhand ☐ Shoulder-width ☐ Wider ☐ Band-strength	Push-Up-Bars ☐ One arm ☐ Shoulder-width ☐	Overhand ☐ Underhand ☐ Shoulder-width ☐ Wider ☐ Band-strength	Push-Up-Bars ☐ One arm ☐ Shoulder-width ☐	

WEEK 23　　from　　　　to

MON	TUE	WED	THU	FRI	SAT	SD
Chin-ups	**Push-ups**	**Chin-ups**	**Push-ups**	**Chin-ups**	**Push-ups**	REST
Repe-titions	Repe-titions	Repe-titions	Repe-titions	Repe-titions	Repe-titions	
Overhand ☐ Underhand ☐ Shoulder-width ☐ Wider ☐ Band-strength	Push-Up-Bars ☐ One arm ☐ Shoulder-width ☐	Overhand ☐ Underhand ☐ Shoulder-width ☐ Wider ☐ Band-strength	Push-Up-Bars ☐ One arm ☐ Shoulder-width ☐	Overhand ☐ Underhand ☐ Shoulder-width ☐ Wider ☐ Band-strength	Push-Up-Bars ☐ One arm ☐ Shoulder-width ☐	REST

WEEK 24　　from　　　　to

MON	TUE	WED	THU	FRI	SAT	SD
Chin-ups	**Push-ups**	**Chin-ups**	**Push-ups**	**Chin-ups**	**Push-ups**	REST
Repe-titions	Repe-titions	Repe-titions	Repe-titions	Repe-titions	Repe-titions	
Overhand ☐ Underhand ☐ Shoulder-width ☐ Wider ☐ Band-strength	Push-Up-Bars ☐ One arm ☐ Shoulder-width ☐	Overhand ☐ Underhand ☐ Shoulder-width ☐ Wider ☐ Band-strength	Push-Up-Bars ☐ One arm ☐ Shoulder-width ☐	Overhand ☐ Underhand ☐ Shoulder-width ☐ Wider ☐ Band-strength	Push-Up-Bars ☐ One arm ☐ Shoulder-width ☐	REST

WEEK 25   from   to

MON	TUE	WED	THU	FRI	SAT	SD
Chin-ups	Push-ups	Chin-ups	Push-ups	Chin-ups	Push-ups	REST
Repe-titions	Repe-titions	Repe-titions	Repe-titions	Repe-titions	Repe-titions	
Overhand ☐ Underhand ☐ Shoulder-width ☐ Wider ☐ Band-strength	Push-Up-Bars ☐ One arm ☐ Shoulder-width ☐	Overhand ☐ Underhand ☐ Shoulder-width ☐ Wider ☐ Band-strength	Push-Up-Bars ☐ One arm ☐ Shoulder-width ☐	Overhand ☐ Underhand ☐ Shoulder-width ☐ Wider ☐ Band-strength	Push-Up-Bars ☐ One arm ☐ Shoulder-width ☐	

WEEK 26   from   to

MON	TUE	WED	THU	FRI	SAT	SD
Chin-ups	Push-ups	Chin-ups	Push-ups	Chin-ups	Push-ups	REST
Repe-titions	Repe-titions	Repe-titions	Repe-titions	Repe-titions	Repe-titions	
Overhand ☐ Underhand ☐ Shoulder-width ☐ Wider ☐ Band-strength	Push-Up-Bars ☐ One arm ☐ Shoulder-width ☐	Overhand ☐ Underhand ☐ Shoulder-width ☐ Wider ☐ Band-strength	Push-Up-Bars ☐ One arm ☐ Shoulder-width ☐	Overhand ☐ Underhand ☐ Shoulder-width ☐ Wider ☐ Band-strength	Push-Up-Bars ☐ One arm ☐ Shoulder-width ☐	

WEEK 27   from   to

MON	TUE	WED	THU	FRI	SAT	SD
Chin-ups	Push-ups	Chin-ups	Push-ups	Chin-ups	Push-ups	
Repe-titions	Repe-titions	Repe-titions	Repe-titions	Repe-titions	Repe-titions	
Overhand ☐ Underhand ☐ Shoulder-width ☐ Wider ☐ Band-strength	Push-Up-Bars ☐ One arm ☐ Shoulder-width ☐	Overhand ☐ Underhand ☐ Shoulder-width ☐ Wider ☐ Band-strength	Push-Up-Bars ☐ One arm ☐ Shoulder-width ☐	Overhand ☐ Underhand ☐ Shoulder-width ☐ Wider ☐ Band-strength	Push-Up-Bars ☐ One arm ☐ Shoulder-width ☐	REST

WEEK 28   from   to

MON	TUE	WED	THU	FRI	SAT	SD
Chin-ups	Push-ups	Chin-ups	Push-ups	Chin-ups	Push-ups	
Repe-titions	Repe-titions	Repe-titions	Repe-titions	Repe-titions	Repe-titions	
Overhand ☐ Underhand ☐ Shoulder-width ☐ Wider ☐ Band-strength	Push-Up-Bars ☐ One arm ☐ Shoulder-width ☐	Overhand ☐ Underhand ☐ Shoulder-width ☐ Wider ☐ Band-strength	Push-Up-Bars ☐ One arm ☐ Shoulder-width ☐	Overhand ☐ Underhand ☐ Shoulder-width ☐ Wider ☐ Band-strength	Push-Up-Bars ☐ One arm ☐ Shoulder-width ☐	REST

WEEK 29   from   to

MON	TUE	WED	THU	FRI	SAT	SD
Chin-ups	**Push-ups**	**Chin-ups**	**Push-ups**	**Chin-ups**	**Push-ups**	
Repe-titions	Repe-titions	Repe-titions	Repe-titions	Repe-titions	Repe-titions	
Overhand ☐ Underhand ☐ Shoulder-width ☐ Wider ☐ Band-strength	Push-Up-Bars ☐ One arm ☐ Shoulder-width ☐	Overhand ☐ Underhand ☐ Shoulder-width ☐ Wider ☐ Band-strength	Push-Up-Bars ☐ One arm ☐ Shoulder-width ☐	Overhand ☐ Underhand ☐ Shoulder-width ☐ Wider ☐ Band-strength	Push-Up-Bars ☐ One arm ☐ Shoulder-width ☐	REST

WEEK 30   from   to

MON	TUE	WED	THU	FRI	SAT	SD
Chin-ups	**Push-ups**	**Chin-ups**	**Push-ups**	**Chin-ups**	**Push-ups**	
Repe-titions	Repe-titions	Repe-titions	Repe-titions	Repe-titions	Repe-titions	
Overhand ☐ Underhand ☐ Shoulder-width ☐ Wider ☐ Band-strength	Push-Up-Bars ☐ One arm ☐ Shoulder-width ☐	Overhand ☐ Underhand ☐ Shoulder-width ☐ Wider ☐ Band-strength	Push-Up-Bars ☐ One arm ☐ Shoulder-width ☐	Overhand ☐ Underhand ☐ Shoulder-width ☐ Wider ☐ Band-strength	Push-Up-Bars ☐ One arm ☐ Shoulder-width ☐	REST

WEEK 31   from   to

MON	TUE	WED	THU	FRI	SAT	SD
Chin-ups	Push-ups	Chin-ups	Push-ups	Chin-ups	Push-ups	REST
Repe-titions	Repe-titions	Repe-titions	Repe-titions	Repe-titions	Repe-titions	
Overhand ☐ Underhand ☐ Shoulder-width ☐ Wider ☐ Band-strength	Push-Up-Bars ☐ One arm ☐ Shoulder-width ☐	Overhand ☐ Underhand ☐ Shoulder-width ☐ Wider ☐ Band-strength	Push-Up-Bars ☐ One arm ☐ Shoulder-width ☐	Overhand ☐ Underhand ☐ Shoulder-width ☐ Wider ☐ Band-strength	Push-Up-Bars ☐ One arm ☐ Shoulder-width ☐	

WEEK 32   from   to

MON	TUE	WED	THU	FRI	SAT	SD
Chin-ups	Push-ups	Chin-ups	Push-ups	Chin-ups	Push-ups	REST
Repe-titions	Repe-titions	Repe-titions	Repe-titions	Repe-titions	Repe-titions	
Overhand ☐ Underhand ☐ Shoulder-width ☐ Wider ☐ Band-strength	Push-Up-Bars ☐ One arm ☐ Shoulder-width ☐	Overhand ☐ Underhand ☐ Shoulder-width ☐ Wider ☐ Band-strength	Push-Up-Bars ☐ One arm ☐ Shoulder-width ☐	Overhand ☐ Underhand ☐ Shoulder-width ☐ Wider ☐ Band-strength	Push-Up-Bars ☐ One arm ☐ Shoulder-width ☐	

WEEK 33   from   to

MON	TUE	WED	THU	FRI	SAT	SD
Chin-ups	Push-ups	Chin-ups	Push-ups	Chin-ups	Push-ups	
Repetitions	Repetitions	Repetitions	Repetitions	Repetitions	Repetitions	
Overhand ☐ Underhand ☐ Shoulder-width ☐ Wider ☐ Band-strength	Push-Up-Bars ☐ One arm ☐ Shoulder-width ☐	Overhand ☐ Underhand ☐ Shoulder-width ☐ Wider ☐ Band-strength	Push-Up-Bars ☐ One arm ☐ Shoulder-width ☐	Overhand ☐ Underhand ☐ Shoulder-width ☐ Wider ☐ Band-strength	Push-Up-Bars ☐ One arm ☐ Shoulder-width ☐	REST

WEEK 34   from   to

MON	TUE	WED	THU	FRI	SAT	SD
Chin-ups	Push-ups	Chin-ups	Push-ups	Chin-ups	Push-ups	
Repetitions	Repetitions	Repetitions	Repetitions	Repetitions	Repetitions	
Overhand ☐ Underhand ☐ Shoulder-width ☐ Wider ☐ Band-strength	Push-Up-Bars ☐ One arm ☐ Shoulder-width ☐	Overhand ☐ Underhand ☐ Shoulder-width ☐ Wider ☐ Band-strength	Push-Up-Bars ☐ One arm ☐ Shoulder-width ☐	Overhand ☐ Underhand ☐ Shoulder-width ☐ Wider ☐ Band-strength	Push-Up-Bars ☐ One arm ☐ Shoulder-width ☐	REST

WEEK 35   from   to

MON	TUE	WED	THU	FRI	SAT	SD
Chin-ups	**Push-ups**	**Chin-ups**	**Push-ups**	**Chin-ups**	**Push-ups**	REST
Repetitions	Repetitions	Repetitions	Repetitions	Repetitions	Repetitions	
Overhand ☐ Underhand ☐ Shoulder-width ☐ Wider ☐ Band-strength	Push-Up-Bars ☐ One arm ☐ Shoulder-width ☐	Overhand ☐ Underhand ☐ Shoulder-width ☐ Wider ☐ Band-strength	Push-Up-Bars ☐ One arm ☐ Shoulder-width ☐	Overhand ☐ Underhand ☐ Shoulder-width ☐ Wider ☐ Band-strength	Push-Up-Bars ☐ One arm ☐ Shoulder-width ☐	

WEEK 36   from   to

MON	TUE	WED	THU	FRI	SAT	SD
Chin-ups	**Push-ups**	**Chin-ups**	**Push-ups**	**Chin-ups**	**Push-ups**	REST
Repetitions	Repetitions	Repetitions	Repetitions	Repetitions	Repetitions	
Overhand ☐ Underhand ☐ Shoulder-width ☐ Wider ☐ Band-strength	Push-Up-Bars ☐ One arm ☐ Shoulder-width ☐	Overhand ☐ Underhand ☐ Shoulder-width ☐ Wider ☐ Band-strength	Push-Up-Bars ☐ One arm ☐ Shoulder-width ☐	Overhand ☐ Underhand ☐ Shoulder-width ☐ Wider ☐ Band-strength	Push-Up-Bars ☐ One arm ☐ Shoulder-width ☐	

WEEK 37   from   to

MON	TUE	WED	THU	FRI	SAT	SD
Chin-ups	Push-ups	Chin-ups	Push-ups	Chin-ups	Push-ups	REST
Repe-titions	Repe-titions	Repe-titions	Repe-titions	Repe-titions	Repe-titions	
Overhand ☐ Underhand ☐ Shoulder-width ☐ Wider ☐ Band-strength	Push-Up-Bars ☐ One arm ☐ Shoulder-width ☐	Overhand ☐ Underhand ☐ Shoulder-width ☐ Wider ☐ Band-strength	Push-Up-Bars ☐ One arm ☐ Shoulder-width ☐	Overhand ☐ Underhand ☐ Shoulder-width ☐ Wider ☐ Band-strength	Push-Up-Bars ☐ One arm ☐ Shoulder-width ☐	

WEEK 38   from   to

MON	TUE	WED	THU	FRI	SAT	SD
Chin-ups	Push-ups	Chin-ups	Push-ups	Chin-ups	Push-ups	REST
Repe-titions	Repe-titions	Repe-titions	Repe-titions	Repe-titions	Repe-titions	
Overhand ☐ Underhand ☐ Shoulder-width ☐ Wider ☐ Band-strength	Push-Up-Bars ☐ One arm ☐ Shoulder-width ☐	Overhand ☐ Underhand ☐ Shoulder-width ☐ Wider ☐ Band-strength	Push-Up-Bars ☐ One arm ☐ Shoulder-width ☐	Overhand ☐ Underhand ☐ Shoulder-width ☐ Wider ☐ Band-strength	Push-Up-Bars ☐ One arm ☐ Shoulder-width ☐	

WEEK 39   from   to

MON	TUE	WED	THU	FRI	SAT	SD
Chin-ups	**Push-ups**	**Chin-ups**	**Push-ups**	**Chin-ups**	**Push-ups**	
Repe-titions	Repe-titions	Repe-titions	Repe-titions	Repe-titions	Repe-titions	
Overhand ☐ Underhand ☐ Shoulder-width ☐ Wider ☐ Band-strength	Push-Up-Bars ☐ One arm ☐ Shoulder-width ☐	Overhand ☐ Underhand ☐ Shoulder-width ☐ Wider ☐ Band-strength	Push-Up-Bars ☐ One arm ☐ Shoulder-width ☐	Overhand ☐ Underhand ☐ Shoulder-width ☐ Wider ☐ Band-strength	Push-Up-Bars ☐ One arm ☐ Shoulder-width ☐	REST

WEEK 40   from   to

MON	TUE	WED	THU	FRI	SAT	SD
Chin-ups	**Push-ups**	**Chin-ups**	**Push-ups**	**Chin-ups**	**Push-ups**	
Repe-titions	Repe-titions	Repe-titions	Repe-titions	Repe-titions	Repe-titions	
Overhand ☐ Underhand ☐ Shoulder-width ☐ Wider ☐ Band-strength	Push-Up-Bars ☐ One arm ☐ Shoulder-width ☐	Overhand ☐ Underhand ☐ Shoulder-width ☐ Wider ☐ Band-strength	Push-Up-Bars ☐ One arm ☐ Shoulder-width ☐	Overhand ☐ Underhand ☐ Shoulder-width ☐ Wider ☐ Band-strength	Push-Up-Bars ☐ One arm ☐ Shoulder-width ☐	REST

WEEK 41   from   to

MON	TUE	WED	THU	FRI	SAT	SD
Chin-ups	**Push-ups**	**Chin-ups**	**Push-ups**	**Chin-ups**	**Push-ups**	
Repe-titions	Repe-titions	Repe-titions	Repe-titions	Repe-titions	Repe-titions	
Overhand ☐ Underhand ☐ Shoulder-width ☐ Wider ☐ Band-strength	Push-Up-Bars ☐ One arm ☐ Shoulder-width ☐	Overhand ☐ Underhand ☐ Shoulder-width ☐ Wider ☐ Band-strength	Push-Up-Bars ☐ One arm ☐ Shoulder-width ☐	Overhand ☐ Underhand ☐ Shoulder-width ☐ Wider ☐ Band-strength	Push-Up-Bars ☐ One arm ☐ Shoulder-width ☐	REST

WEEK 42   from   to

MON	TUE	WED	THU	FRI	SAT	SD
Chin-ups	**Push-ups**	**Chin-ups**	**Push-ups**	**Chin-ups**	**Push-ups**	
Repe-titions	Repe-titions	Repe-titions	Repe-titions	Repe-titions	Repe-titions	
Overhand ☐ Underhand ☐ Shoulder-width ☐ Wider ☐ Band-strength	Push-Up-Bars ☐ One arm ☐ Shoulder-width ☐	Overhand ☐ Underhand ☐ Shoulder-width ☐ Wider ☐ Band-strength	Push-Up-Bars ☐ One arm ☐ Shoulder-width ☐	Overhand ☐ Underhand ☐ Shoulder-width ☐ Wider ☐ Band-strength	Push-Up-Bars ☐ One arm ☐ Shoulder-width ☐	REST

WEEK 43   from   to

MON	TUE	WED	THU	FRI	SAT	SD
Chin-ups	Push-ups	Chin-ups	Push-ups	Chin-ups	Push-ups	REST
Repe-titions	Repe-titions	Repe-titions	Repe-titions	Repe-titions	Repe-titions	
Overhand ☐ Underhand ☐ Shoulder-width ☐ Wider ☐ Band-strength	Push-Up-Bars ☐ One arm ☐ Shoulder-width ☐	Overhand ☐ Underhand ☐ Shoulder-width ☐ Wider ☐ Band-strength	Push-Up-Bars ☐ One arm ☐ Shoulder-width ☐	Overhand ☐ Underhand ☐ Shoulder-width ☐ Wider ☐ Band-strength	Push-Up-Bars ☐ One arm ☐ Shoulder-width ☐	

WEEK 44   from   to

MON	TUE	WED	THU	FRI	SAT	SD
Chin-ups	Push-ups	Chin-ups	Push-ups	Chin-ups	Push-ups	REST
Repe-titions	Repe-titions	Repe-titions	Repe-titions	Repe-titions	Repe-titions	
Overhand ☐ Underhand ☐ Shoulder-width ☐ Wider ☐ Band-strength	Push-Up-Bars ☐ One arm ☐ Shoulder-width ☐	Overhand ☐ Underhand ☐ Shoulder-width ☐ Wider ☐ Band-strength	Push-Up-Bars ☐ One arm ☐ Shoulder-width ☐	Overhand ☐ Underhand ☐ Shoulder-width ☐ Wider ☐ Band-strength	Push-Up-Bars ☐ One arm ☐ Shoulder-width ☐	

WEEK 45   from   to

MON	TUE	WED	THU	FRI	SAT	SD
Chin-ups	Push-ups	Chin-ups	Push-ups	Chin-ups	Push-ups	REST
Repetitions	Repetitions	Repetitions	Repetitions	Repetitions	Repetitions	
Overhand ☐ Underhand ☐ Shoulder-width ☐ Wider ☐ Band-strength	Push-Up-Bars ☐ One arm ☐ Shoulder-width ☐	Overhand ☐ Underhand ☐ Shoulder-width ☐ Wider ☐ Band-strength	Push-Up-Bars ☐ One arm ☐ Shoulder-width ☐	Overhand ☐ Underhand ☐ Shoulder-width ☐ Wider ☐ Band-strength	Push-Up-Bars ☐ One arm ☐ Shoulder-width ☐	

WEEK 46   from   to

MON	TUE	WED	THU	FRI	SAT	SD
Chin-ups	Push-ups	Chin-ups	Push-ups	Chin-ups	Push-ups	REST
Repetitions	Repetitions	Repetitions	Repetitions	Repetitions	Repetitions	
Overhand ☐ Underhand ☐ Shoulder-width ☐ Wider ☐ Band-strength	Push-Up-Bars ☐ One arm ☐ Shoulder-width ☐	Overhand ☐ Underhand ☐ Shoulder-width ☐ Wider ☐ Band-strength	Push-Up-Bars ☐ One arm ☐ Shoulder-width ☐	Overhand ☐ Underhand ☐ Shoulder-width ☐ Wider ☐ Band-strength	Push-Up-Bars ☐ One arm ☐ Shoulder-width ☐	

WEEK 47   from   to

MON	TUE	WED	THU	FRI	SAT	SD
Chin-ups	**Push-ups**	**Chin-ups**	**Push-ups**	**Chin-ups**	**Push-ups**	
Repetitions	Repetitions	Repetitions	Repetitions	Repetitions	Repetitions	
Overhand ☐ Underhand ☐ Shoulder-width ☐ Wider ☐ Band-strength	Push-Up-Bars ☐ One arm ☐ Shoulder-width ☐	Overhand ☐ Underhand ☐ Shoulder-width ☐ Wider ☐ Band-strength	Push-Up-Bars ☐ One arm ☐ Shoulder-width ☐	Overhand ☐ Underhand ☐ Shoulder-width ☐ Wider ☐ Band-strength	Push-Up-Bars ☐ One arm ☐ Shoulder-width ☐	REST

WEEK 48   from   to

MON	TUE	WED	THU	FRI	SAT	SD
Chin-ups	**Push-ups**	**Chin-ups**	**Push-ups**	**Chin-ups**	**Push-ups**	
Repetitions	Repetitions	Repetitions	Repetitions	Repetitions	Repetitions	
Overhand ☐ Underhand ☐ Shoulder-width ☐ Wider ☐ Band-strength	Push-Up-Bars ☐ One arm ☐ Shoulder-width ☐	Overhand ☐ Underhand ☐ Shoulder-width ☐ Wider ☐ Band-strength	Push-Up-Bars ☐ One arm ☐ Shoulder-width ☐	Overhand ☐ Underhand ☐ Shoulder-width ☐ Wider ☐ Band-strength	Push-Up-Bars ☐ One arm ☐ Shoulder-width ☐	REST

WEEK 49   from   to

MON	TUE	WED	THU	FRI	SAT	SD
Chin-ups	Push-ups	Chin-ups	Push-ups	Chin-ups	Push-ups	
Repe-titions	Repe-titions	Repe-titions	Repe-titions	Repe-titions	Repe-titions	
Overhand ☐ Underhand ☐ Shoulder-width ☐ Wider ☐ Band-strength	Push-Up-Bars ☐ One arm ☐ Shoulder-width ☐	Overhand ☐ Underhand ☐ Shoulder-width ☐ Wider ☐ Band-strength	Push-Up-Bars ☐ One arm ☐ Shoulder-width ☐	Overhand ☐ Underhand ☐ Shoulder-width ☐ Wider ☐ Band-strength	Push-Up-Bars ☐ One arm ☐ Shoulder-width ☐	REST

WEEK 50   from   to

MON	TUE	WED	THU	FRI	SAT	SD
Chin-ups	Push-ups	Chin-ups	Push-ups	Chin-ups	Push-ups	
Repe-titions	Repe-titions	Repe-titions	Repe-titions	Repe-titions	Repe-titions	
Overhand ☐ Underhand ☐ Shoulder-width ☐ Wider ☐ Band-strength	Push-Up-Bars ☐ One arm ☐ Shoulder-width ☐	Overhand ☐ Underhand ☐ Shoulder-width ☐ Wider ☐ Band-strength	Push-Up-Bars ☐ One arm ☐ Shoulder-width ☐	Overhand ☐ Underhand ☐ Shoulder-width ☐ Wider ☐ Band-strength	Push-Up-Bars ☐ One arm ☐ Shoulder-width ☐	REST

WEEK 51   from   to

MON	TUE	WED	THU	FRI	SAT	SD
Chin-ups	**Push-ups**	**Chin-ups**	**Push-ups**	**Chin-ups**	**Push-ups**	REST
Repetitions	Repetitions	Repetitions	Repetitions	Repetitions	Repetitions	
Overhand ☐ Underhand ☐ Shoulder-width ☐ Wider ☐ Band-strength	Push-Up-Bars ☐ One arm ☐ Shoulder-width ☐	Overhand ☐ Underhand ☐ Shoulder-width ☐ Wider ☐ Band-strength	Push-Up-Bars ☐ One arm ☐ Shoulder-width ☐	Overhand ☐ Underhand ☐ Shoulder-width ☐ Wider ☐ Band-strength	Push-Up-Bars ☐ One arm ☐ Shoulder-width ☐	

WEEK 52   from   to

MON	TUE	WED	THU	FRI	SAT	SD
Chin-ups	**Push-ups**	**Chin-ups**	**Push-ups**	**Chin-ups**	**Push-ups**	REST
Repetitions	Repetitions	Repetitions	Repetitions	Repetitions	Repetitions	
Overhand ☐ Underhand ☐ Shoulder-width ☐ Wider ☐ Band-strength	Push-Up-Bars ☐ One arm ☐ Shoulder-width ☐	Overhand ☐ Underhand ☐ Shoulder-width ☐ Wider ☐ Band-strength	Push-Up-Bars ☐ One arm ☐ Shoulder-width ☐	Overhand ☐ Underhand ☐ Shoulder-width ☐ Wider ☐ Band-strength	Push-Up-Bars ☐ One arm ☐ Shoulder-width ☐	

Bibliography

1. Punnet, Laura et al. (2005). Estimating the Global Burden of Low Back Pain Attributable to Combined Occupational Exposures; in: American Journal of Industrial Medicine, Vol. 48 (6), S. 459–469

2. Global Burden of Disease, Injury Incidence, Prevalence Collaborators. Global, regional, and national incidence, prevalence, and years lived with disability for 310 diseases and injuries, 1990–2015: a systematic analysis for the Global Burden of Disease Study 2015. In: The Lancet 2016

3. Voermans, Sabine u. a. Beweg Dich Deutschland! TK-Bewegungsstudie 2016

4. George, Bill (2015). Discover Your True North

5. Cialdini, Robert (2006). Influence: The Psychology of Persuasion

6. Barney, Jay (1991). Firm Resources and Sustained Competitive Advantage; in: Journal of Management, Vol. 17 (1), S. 99–120

7. Ericsson, Anders (2016). Peak: Secrets from the New Science of Expertise

8. Koch, Richard (1999). The 80/20 Principle, Expanded and Updated: The Secret to Achieving More with Less

9. Einstein, Albert (2009/1916). Über die spezielle und die allgemeine Relativitätstheorie

10. King, Martin Luther (1963). Letter from Birmingham Jail

11. Gillen, Jenna und Gibala, Martin (2014). Is high-intensity interval training a time-efficient exercise strategy to improve health and fitness? In: Applied Physiology Nutrition and Metabolism Vol. 39 (3), S. 409–412

12. Kieser, Werner (2015). Ein starker Körper kennt keinen Schmerz: Gesundheitsorientiertes Krafttraining nach der Kieser-Methode

13. Gibala, Mark (2017). The One Minute Workout

14. Kadlec, Daniel und Groeger, David (2020). Athletiktraining in der Sportphysiotherapie: Die besten Übungen für Kraft, Schnelligkeit und Stabilität

15. Diemer, Frank und Sutor, Volker (2017). Praxis der medizinischen Trainingstherapie I: Lendenwirbelsäule, Sakroiliakalgelenk und untere Extremität

16. Zimmermann, Klaus (2002). Gesundheitsorientiertes Muskelkrafttraining: Theorie - Empirie – Praxisorientierung

17. Kotter, John (2012). Leading Change

18. Porter, Michael (2004). Competitive Strategy: Techniques for Analyzing Industries and Competitors

19. Clear, James (2018). Atomic Habits, Tiny Changes Remarkable Results

20. Christensen, Clayton; Allworth, James und Dillon, Karen (2012). How Will You Measure Your Life?

Sources

Photos
Lisa Beller with Lasse Schneider
www.lisabeller.de

Illustrations
S.36 & 63 – schoenski.de
S.29 – Freepik.com @dooder

ABOUT THE AUTHORS
AXEL DELKER

Axel is a happily married father of two. He runs a medium-sized enterprise with his brother and does volunteer work in his hometown. A sports fan with a degree in business administration, he has found his own way of keeping in shape amid a full life all the fuller for its many obligations.

LAURA SCHÖFFEL

Laura has been an editorial journalist at a daily newspaper for several years. As a mother of three she lives with her husband close to Frankfurt, Germany. Her whole life Laura has been enthusiastic about horseback riding and for which a strong back always has been an important prerequisite.

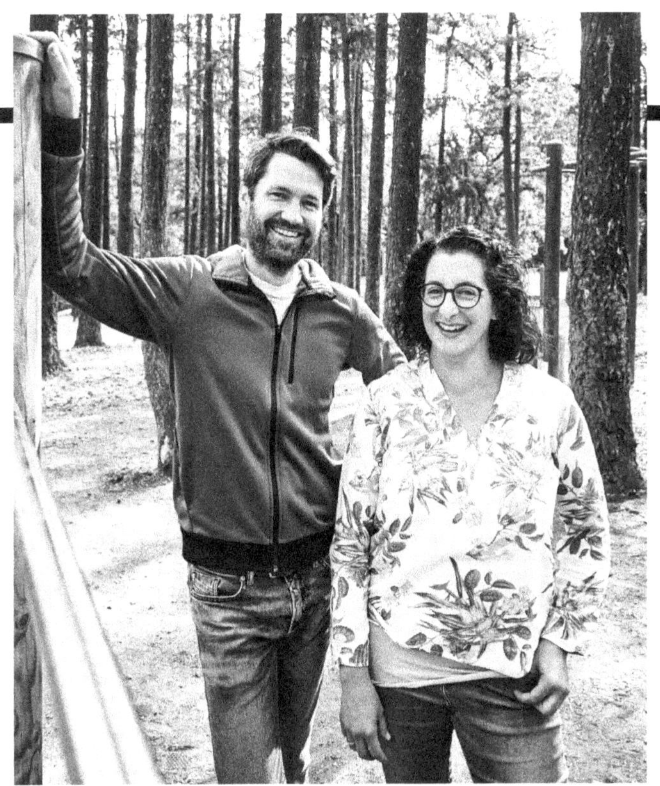

JETZT DU!